INSTANT FITNESS: THE SHAOLIN

KUNG FU

WORKOUT

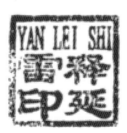

WRITTEN BY SHIFU YAN LEI
PHOTOGRAPHY BY MANUEL VASON

YAN LEI

Published by Yan Lei Press
www.shifuyanlei.co.uk
Text copyright © Shifu Yan Lei
Photographic copyright © Manuel Vason

First published September 2015

Photos taken on location at the Huangshan Mountain,
the Shaolin Temple, and Shaolin Village, China.

ISBN: 978-0-9563101-9-4
A catalogue record of this book is available from
the British Library.
Printed and bound in China.

CREDITS
Photography by Manuel Vason,
www.manuelvason.com
Book design by Andrew Egan and Amy Gustantino, Coolgrayseven,
www.coolgrayseven.com
Martial Arts Technical Advisor: Shifu Yang Hong Zhou,
www.yhsz.com

Thank you to all of my students who bought my first book and have continued to email me asking me when they can read this book. Thank you to my master, Shi Xong Jin for giving me the opportunity to train at the Shaolin Temple. Thank you to my brother Shifu Yan Zi and everyone at Shaolin Temple UK in London.

Thank you to Cat Goscovitch for editing and producing this book. This book could never have happened without your persistence and patience.

Thank you to Manuel Vason, your kung fu is your skill as a photographer.

Thank you to Andrew Egan and Amy Gustantino at Coolgrayseven for capturing the meaning of Shaolin and designing such a beautiful book.

Thank you to my kung fu brother Shifu Hong Zhou for his technical support and hospitality.

I'm very fortunate to have a fantastic team who work tirelessly to promote authentic Shaolin. I couldn't do it without them. The director of my Shaolin Warrior series of DVDs and my first feature film, The Turtle And The Sea, Marek Budzynski. And thank you to Marcus Taylor at www.taylorthomas.co.uk for designing my website and DVD covers.

And finally thank you to you, my loyal students around the world. We have never met but you continue to train with me and put your support and trust in me. I hope that I teach you well.

I dedicate this book to my oldest sister who has just started practicing Shaolin Kung Fu in her fifties.

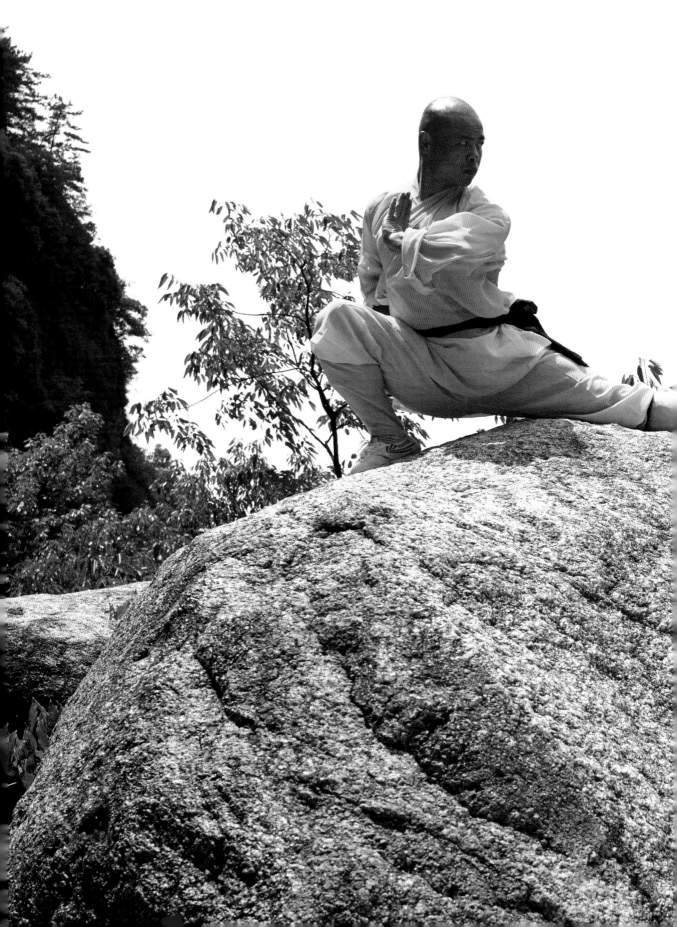

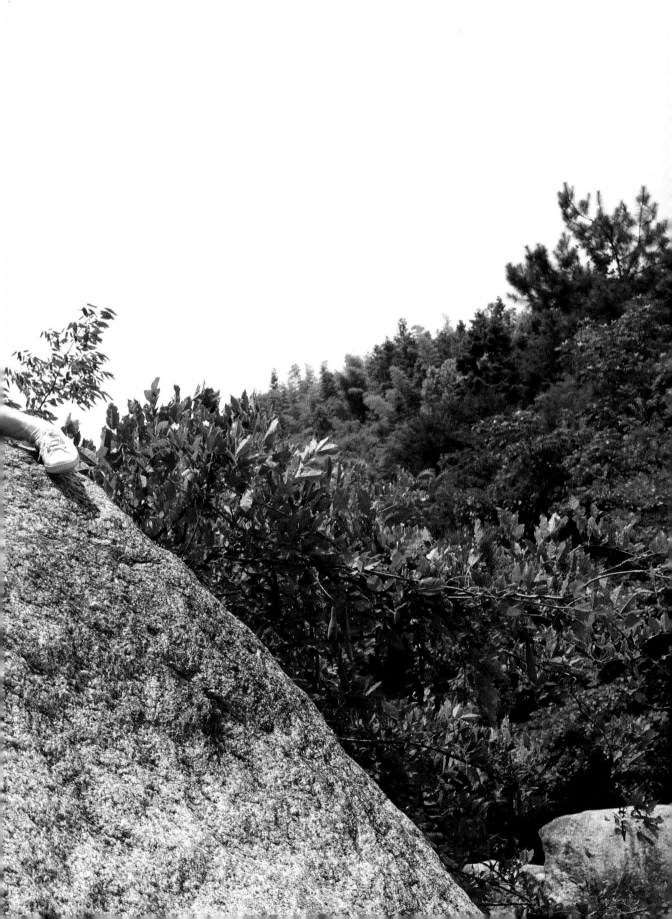

PREFACE

I'm writing this on top of one of the Song Shan Mountains in Henan Province, China, just a few kilometres from the busy Shaolin Temple. I'm alone on the mountain apart from the sound of birds, insects, and a cuckoo calling from the forest below. My Shaolin Summer Camp Students are running on the mountain opposite, preparing for their morning training session.

Being here reminds me of where Shaolin originates. However it's not where we are in terms of location; it's where we are in terms of our heart and mind. Whether I'm on a mountain or in the centre of busy London I'll always find a place to train. Shaolin Kung Fu is my life.

Helping people gain greater fitness, wellness and happiness is my goal in life.

At the Shaolin Temple we train in Kung Fu and Qigong because it contains all the components in one fully integrated unit for health and fitness. This is the reason I wrote my first book, Instant Health: The Shaolin Qigong Workout For Longevity. If you haven't done any exercise for along time then you can start with my first book before moving onto this one.

This book doesn't teach any fighting. It teaches you how to move your body, how to develop your muscles, your tendons, and most importantly, your mind. I've included one very traditional Shaolin form. In the temple this is for high-level martial artists only. This form is like fighting as it consists of footwork, block and attack.

Everything in this book is easy to learn but it's not easy to make good. The goal is not for you to become perfect. The goal is for you to use these exercises to transform your body and your life. You don't need to go to the gym and you don't need any equipment; you can do all of the exercises in your home on the size of a yoga mat.

I hope that wherever you are, through doing these exercises you will enter the Shaolin Zone and experience the peace of being on top of the Song Shan Mountains.

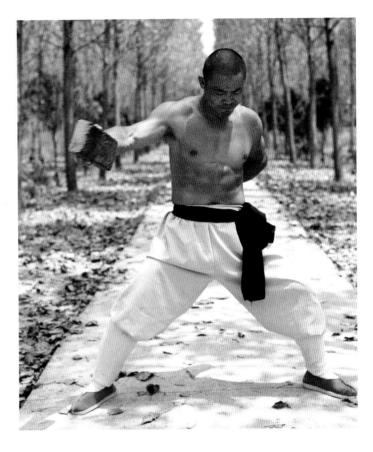

A HAPPY LIFE NEEDS A HEALTHY BODY AND A HEALTHY MIND.

Amituofo,
Shifu Shi Yan Lei

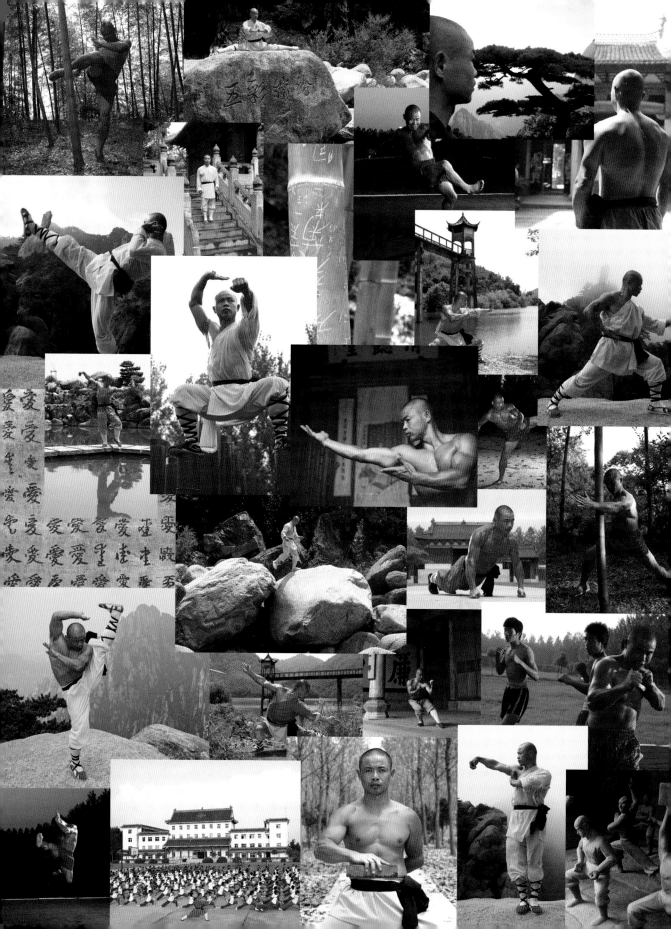

PART ONE

TIME-TESTED TECHNIQUES FOR MIND AND BODY HEALTH

CHAPTER ONE

WHAT IS SHAOLIN KUNG FU?

SHAOLIN KUNG FU ORIGINATES FROM THE SHAOLIN TEMPLE OF ZEN IN CHINA. IT'S A SYSTEM OF MOVEMENTS THAT ARE DESIGNED TO AWAKEN EVERY CELL IN YOUR BODY.

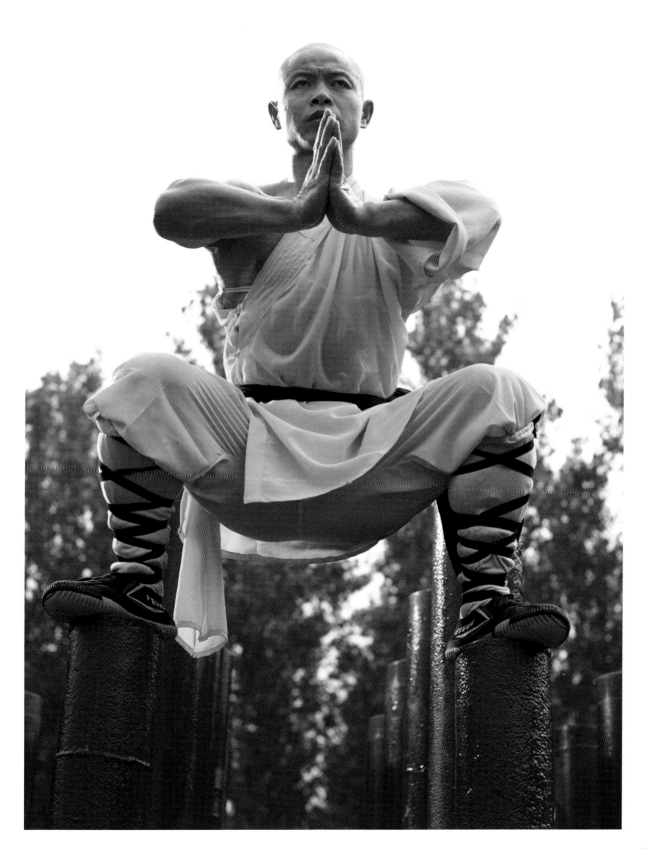

When a student begins to study Shaolin, she not only works her heart aerobically but also inwardly because the movements are done mindfully so that they cultivate her highest qualities of peace and enlightenment.

Shaolin Forms are the only exercise I've come across where every muscle is engaged and we are simultaneously building flexibility, strength, endurance, balance, and power. These ancient forms come from nature, they awaken the body, helping us to let go of our small self and experience a connection with the very fabric of the Universe. They then teach us how to move in our modern life, whether that's carrying our groceries home or climbing the stairs to the subway. Everything becomes part of our training: total mind-body wellness.

Circuit training in the gym consists of squats with weights, press-ups, and lunges. There's nothing wrong with this kind of training but for me, it looks monotonous and doesn't have the gracefulness of Shaolin forms. Shaolin forms work the legs as hard as any squat or lunge but there's a purpose to every movement.

Kung Fu is a Westernised word, the original word is Gong Fu, gong means time, anything that we put our time into is gong fu so if someone is very good at playing the violin then this is their gong fu. Time is one of the reasons why Kung Fu is different from sport. In sport time exists, to the Shaolin Warrior, there is no yesterday, tomorrow or next week. Now is the only thing we have. We always train as if this may be our last training session.

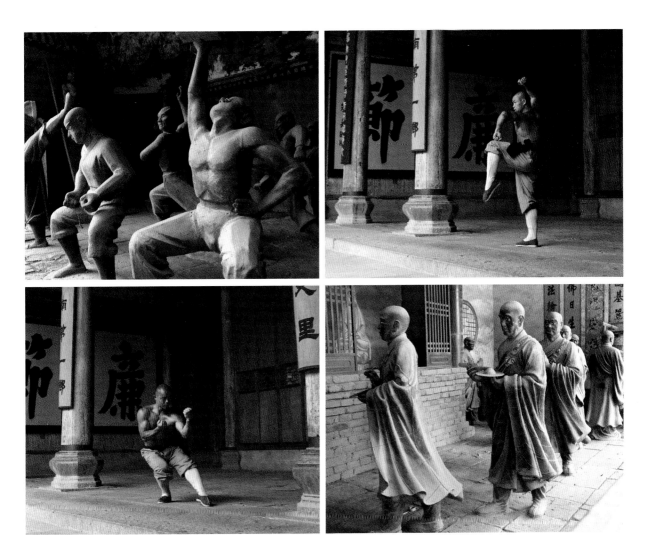

Research has shown that the mind gives up before the body. This means that our body has far more strength and capacity to endure than we give it credit. If you feel that the training is too hard and you want to give up, ask yourself if you have these same feelings in your life. The limits we put on our training are the same limits we put on our life. My master described Shaolin Kung Fu as a fire and our bodies as the metal. Only by putting our self through the fire of hard training can we mould our self into Shaolin Warriors.

The kung fu that I teach in this book is the original Shaolin Kung Fu direct from the temple. My master taught it to me and his master taught it to him and so it goes on in a direct line right back to the founder of Zen, the Bodhidharma. Through reading this book, these precious teachings are being passed on to you. This series of books is a culmination of my twenty years experience of martial arts and the wisdom that I have learned under the instruction of many great masters. Any errors made are not those of my masters or the Shaolin Temple, but my own.

CHAPTER TWO

THE SHAOLIN KUNG FU WORKOUT

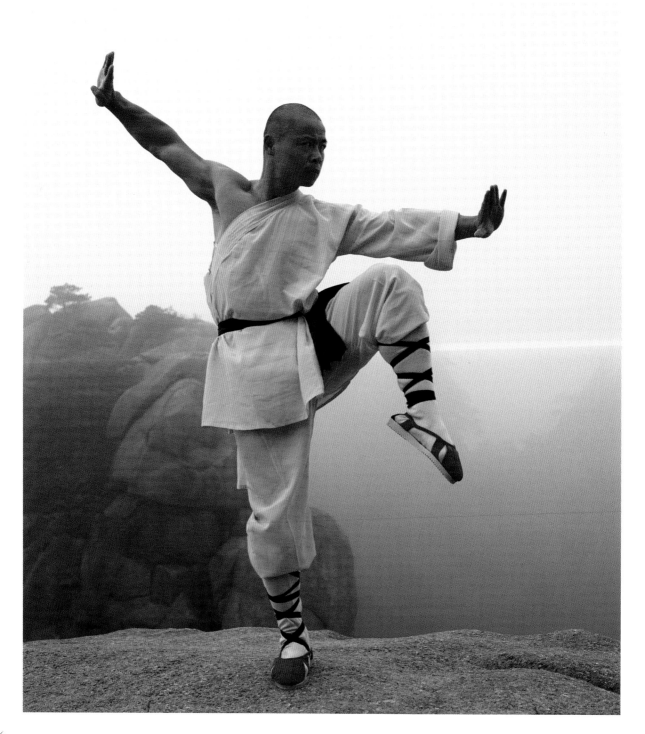

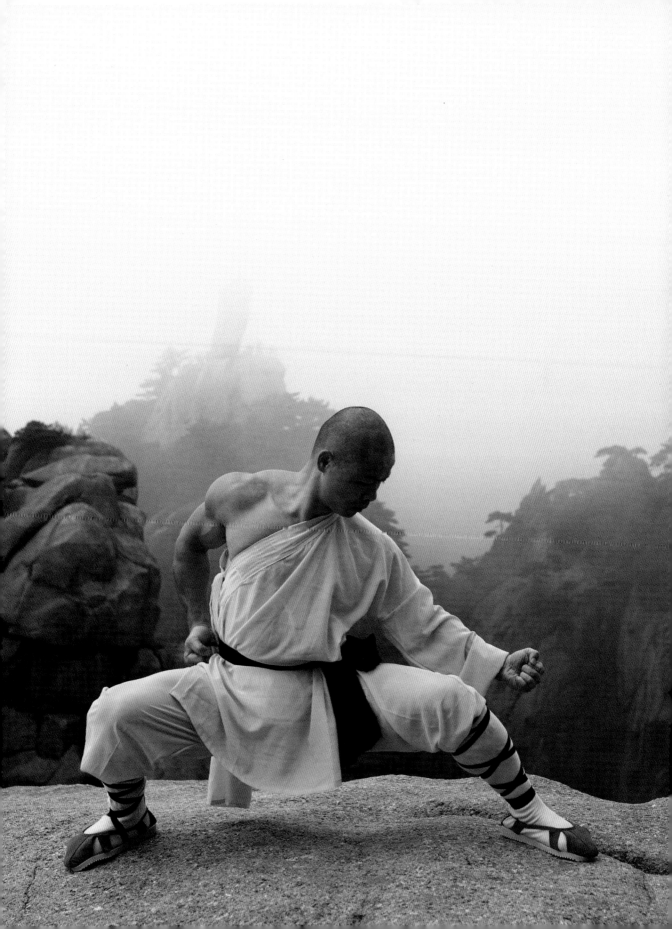

The Shaolin Kung Fu Workout is not a rigid workout but a step-by-step training manual. (You can access some suggested workout program from my website.) When you begin your Shaolin training, it's important that you don't miss a step but you follow the book through to the end. For example, you will never be able to do the forms if you haven't learnt the Five Fundamental Stances and you must master the traditional punches before you move onto the traditional forms.

Take time to learn the fundamentals thoroughly. If you already have my Qigong book then you have a head start, as you will be familiar with the warm up, stretching and Five Fundamental Stances.

At the Shaolin Temple when we run, we run, when we punch, we punch, when we eat, we eat, and when we sleep we sleep. Of course we need to think, but most of our thinking is not useful. Wouldn't it be better if we had more choice over our mind? Wouldn't it be better if we could turn off our thinking like we turn off the TV or switch channels if our thinking is more harmful than helpful? This is the gift our Shaolin training gives us. It's a gift that comes about effortlessly.

Most of the exercises in this book are what every student is taught when they first walk through the gates of the temple. But don't think they're just for beginners. In the temple, when we progress in our training, we still have to attend the beginner's class and go through these drills. I still do these exercises on most days; the only difference is I go through them briefly rather than devoting my whole session to them.

The traditional forms and stances never stop challenging whatever level we are. The Five Fundamental Kicks ensure that our legs and hips stay flexible. If you exercise already, you'll find that the practice of Shaolin will have a positive impact on your chosen sport, increasing your speed, strength and focus. If you have limited time then all you need to do is the exercises in this book coupled with Shaolin Qigong, and this is enough to keep you fit and well for the rest of your life.

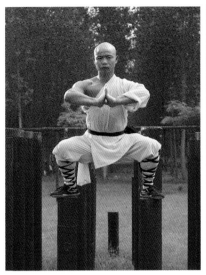
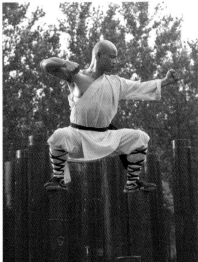
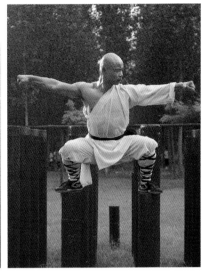
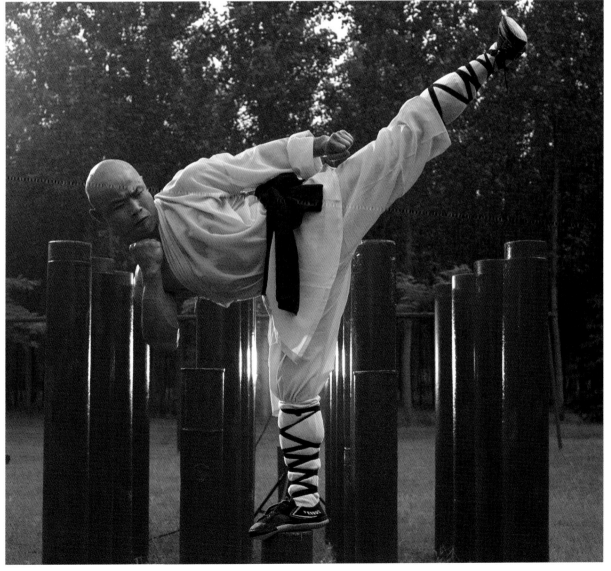

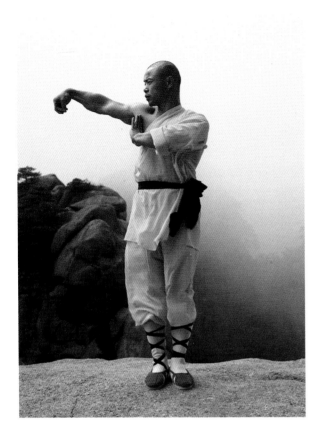
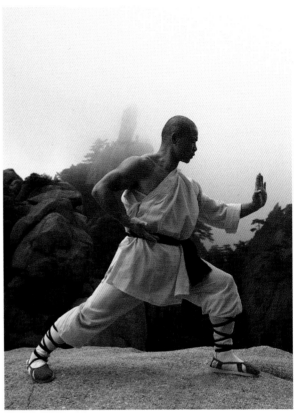
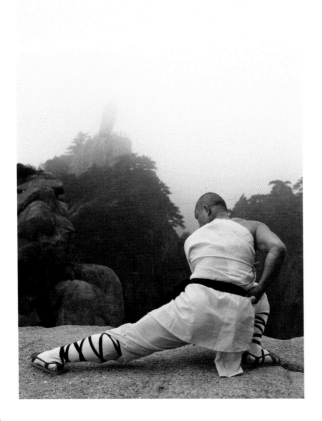
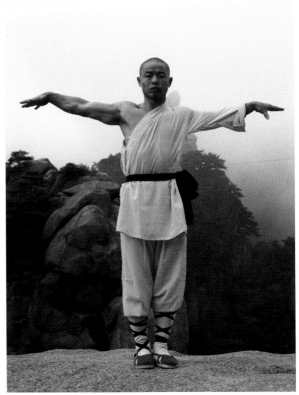

Your Shaolin Workout exercises are also taught in my Shaolin Workout Volume 1, DVD and download, which is available from my website.

YOUR SHAOLIN WORKOUT CONSISTS OF:

– WARM UP
– STRETCHING
– STAMINA TRAINING
– FIVE FUNDAMENTAL KICKS
– FIVE FUNDAMENTAL STANCES
– TRADITIONAL PUNCHES
– TRADITIONAL FORMS
– COOL DOWN WITH SOME QIGONG
  AND QIGONG INSTANT HEALTH MASSAGE.

If you're a martial artist then you need to start your training with a run, and increase in volume as your week goes on, for example, 5k then 7k then 8 k finishing with 10k or run for 5k then do some sprint runs. It's good to vary your pace as you run.

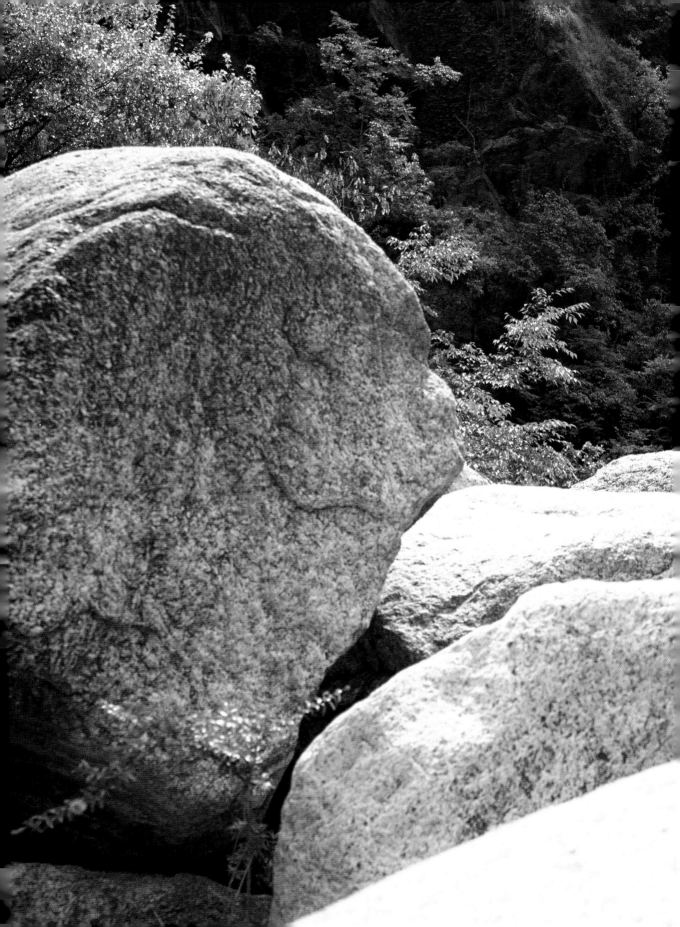

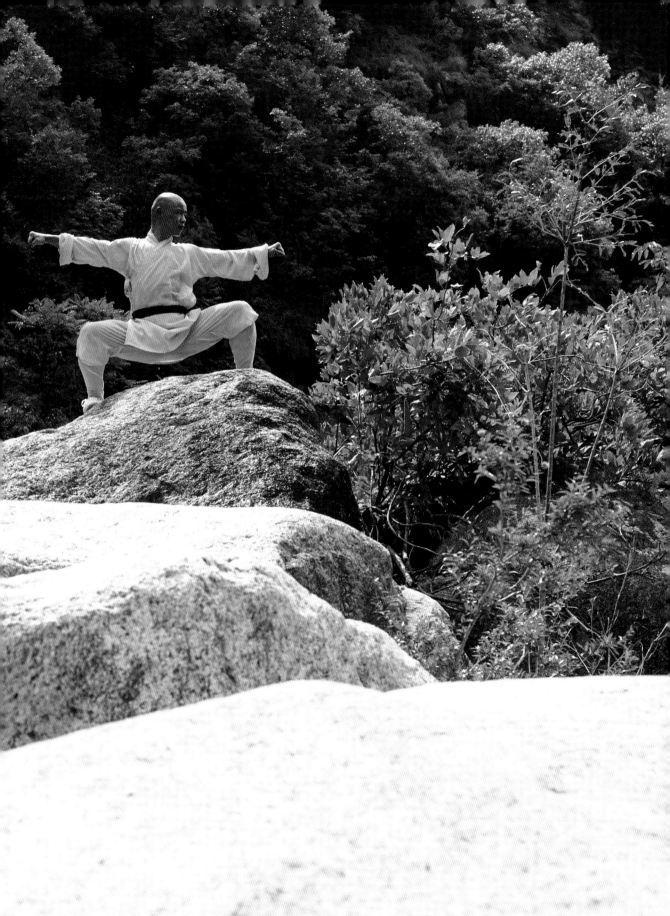

As a martial artist you need to train 6 days a week and for basic fitness you need to train 5 times a week. There are challenges when training alone and I've set up a Facebook group for people who train with my books, DVDs and downloads so that you can support each other. The difficulty is in finding the balance between pushing yourself too hard and not pushing yourself hard enough. If you come for a private session with me, I can read your body and I know what you need. Most people don't push themselves hard enough. It's something you need to experiment with. You need to be challenged but not so challenged that you make yourself sick or injure your body. There should be no pain when you train but there should be muscle ache the next day as you are using muscles you've never used before.

As you get to know the forms, vary the intensity of them. The forms can be done slow like a Qigong form, the better you get the faster you can do the form. Try to video yourself to check if you're doing it correctly or check your form in the mirror. The progression with the Five Fundamental Kicks is how fast and how straight your legs are.

The photos in this book are a guide and inspiration. If you haven't done any exercise before or you are as stiff as a board please don't be discouraged.

You'll get as much benefit from your stretch and stance as I do from mine and you'll be surprised at how flexible and strong you become.

It's important to supplement your kung fu training with Qigong from my Qigong Workout For Longevity book. A bird cannot fly with only one wing. In Shaolin, we say that to be truly balanced, healthy and well, we need to do both Qigong and Kung Fu. We know that our muscles shrink as we get older and our bones can become brittle, exercise can help to prevent this but what about our internal organs? We only think about them when something goes wrong. Qigong oxygenates our internal organs and helps to prevent ill health. Qigong is the reason why, at 42, I still practice as hard as I did when I was 14.

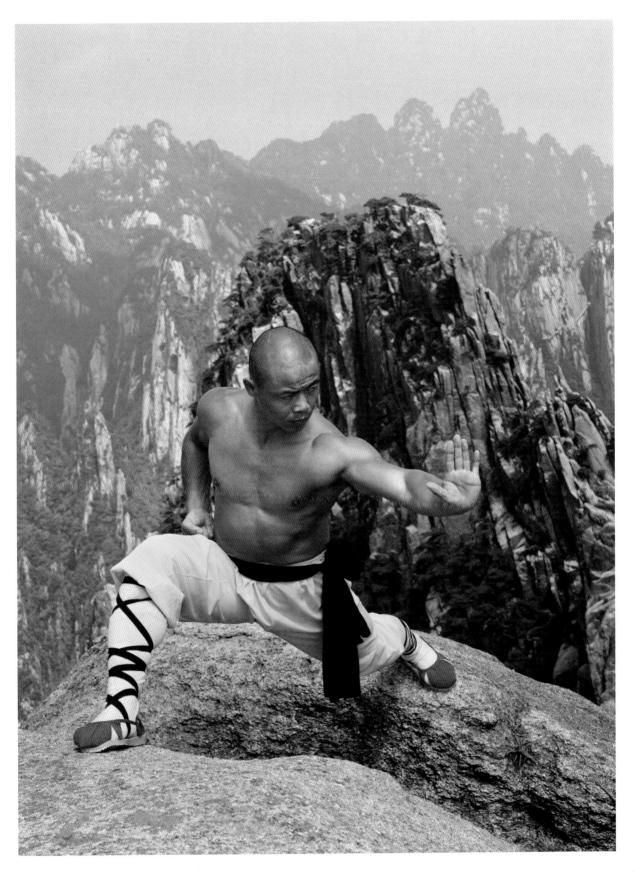

CHAPTER THREE

ZEN: TRAINING THE HEART

"YOUR LIFE IS A ZEN KOAN THAT YOU MUST SOLVE"

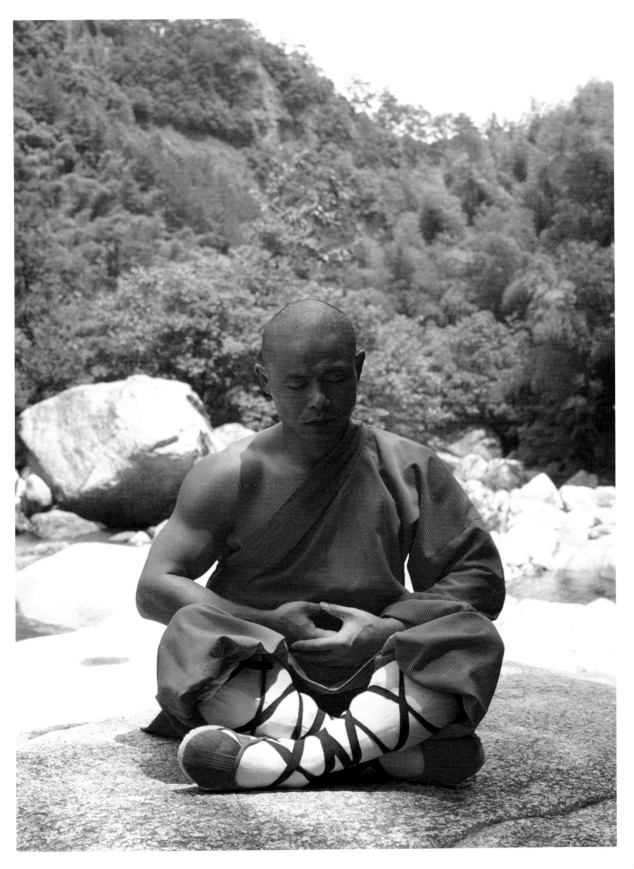

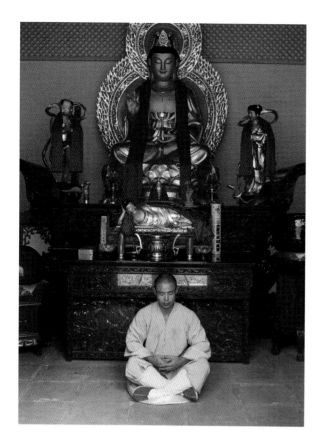 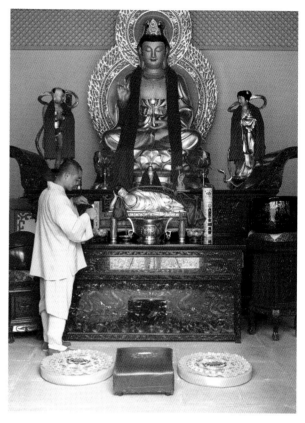

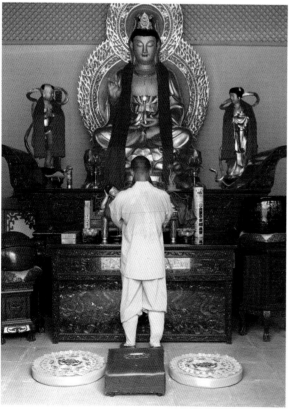 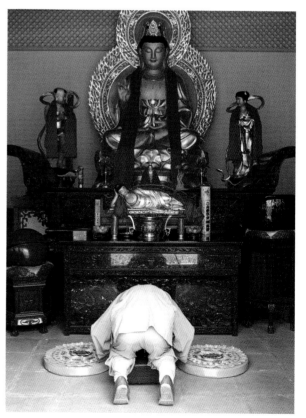

When Bodhidharma arrived in China from India, he found that Buddhism was being studied rather than experienced. Bodhidharma travelled to the Shaolin Temple and started a new school of Buddhism called Zen, Ch'an in Chinese but it can also be translated as The Buddha Heart School.

There is a famous story about a scholar called Eka who went to the temple to see Bodhidharma and ask him to teach him. Bodhidharma didn't turn around. This continued for a week then on the eighth day it started to snow. The next morning, Eka was still kneeling at the gates of the temple, knee deep in snow. Finally Bodhidharma turned and looked at him.

Eka said, "Please teach me," and the Bodhidharma replied, "How can you expect to see the truth? Training with a lazy conceited heart is training in vain." Eka, as proof of his commitment, cut off his left arm and presented it to Bodhidharma. Eka then said, "Please put my heart at ease." Bodhidharma replied, "Put your heart before me and I will put it as ease." Eka said, "My heart doesn't stop for one moment, but I can't find it or get hold of it." Bodhidharma replied, "There, I have put your heart at rest for you."

What does this story mean? The first thing to make clear is that Eka didn't literally cut his arm off. It's a symbol that he released his limited past experiences. It is like the famous story of the student who went to see the Zen master to request teaching. The master invited him for a cup of tea, they sat down and the master picked up the teapot and poured tea into the student's cup and kept pouring until the tea flowed out of the cup and onto the table. The student said, 'Master, what are you doing, my cup is full?" The master replied, "Yes, your cup is full so I can't teach you anything." Eka cutting off his arm was a way of him saying I have emptied my cup and I now have room to receive your teachings.

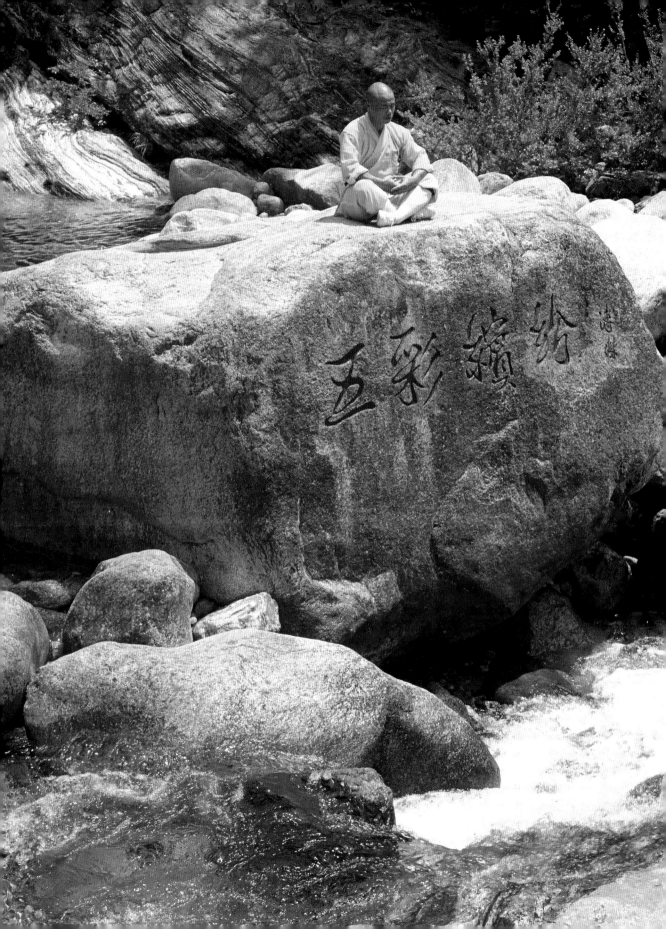

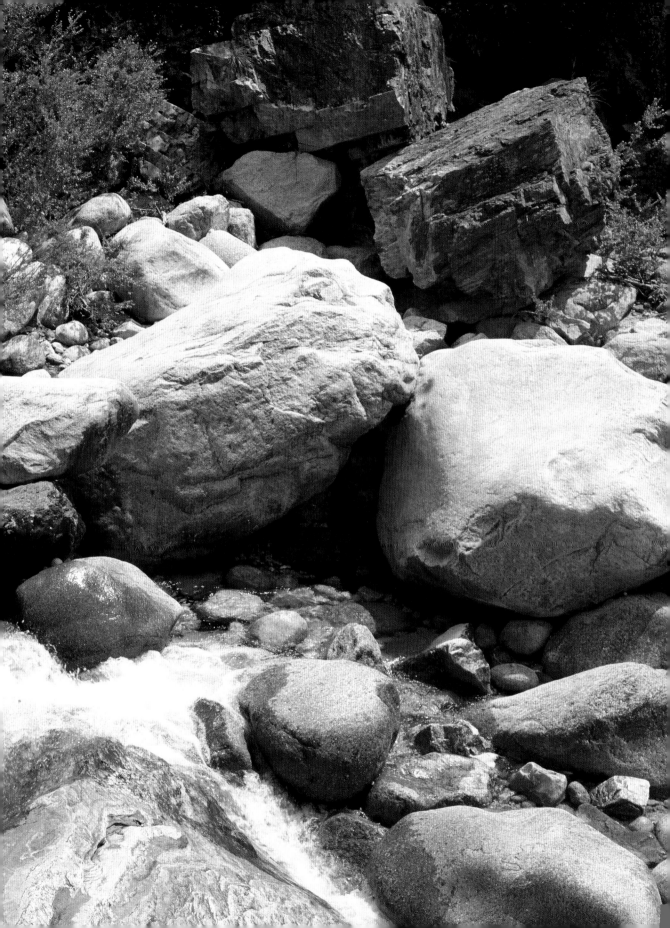

It doesn't matter what religion you practice or whether you practice none at all, we all have the same desire to feel happy, whole and complete. We think if we have a big house or a million pounds or a family or that job we want or that degree or a six-pack then we will be happy. But the only way to complete our self and feel truly happy is by putting our heart at rest, and how do we put our heart at rest? Through understanding the nature of our heart. To understand the nature of our heart is not to study the Buddha as something outside of our self, but to stop looking outside our self for happiness or answers and instead turn our focus onto our own mind so we can see into its true nature.

The Buddha said we need to do two things:

1) TRAIN OUR MIND
2) UNDERSTAND WHO WE ARE

That is all. End of teaching. Sounds easy? In Zen we train our mind in our daily activities. We don't separate; now John is going to sit on a cushion for twenty minutes and he will meditate and be a Buddha but for the rest of his 23 hours and 40 minutes he will be John.

In Zen, we are a Buddha 24 hours a day. And when I say Buddha, please don't be put off by the term Buddha or Buddhist, they are just labels. Buddha simply means awakened one. The historical Buddha awakened to how the world truly is and this gave him everlasting happiness. The Buddha was a normal human being and we are too. We can also do the same as the Buddha. Being awake means we stay present in each moment. This regulates our nervous system, and harmonizes our mind and body.

Most people believe meditation is sitting on a cushion but this is only one type of meditation. I advise my students not to do sitting meditation when they come home from work. Why? Let's say that you have desk job and you've been sitting at your computer all day, your mind has been very active. To then come home and sit on a cushion and expect your mind to calm down will take a great deal of effort. Your body also has needs. We recognise when it needs to eat but many of us have lost the art of listening to the need of our body to be active. If you feel tired be aware that tiredness can come from a body that doesn't move. The best thing you can do after work is train in Shaolin. This is your meditation practice.

Tell yourself, for this one hour I'm going to dedicate myself to my training. You can dedicate your training to someone who is unwell and this strengthens your training. Now you're not just training for yourself, you're training for someone else.

Turn off your phone and anything else that may distract you. Light a candle if you want to the Buddha or whoever inspires you. Begin your Shaolin program. Be aware every time your mind moves from your training but don't get annoyed with yourself. It's pride to expect to be perfect. We think most of the time so it's not so easy to turn it off.

As you move through your Shaolin Workout, you will find that your mind effortlessly begins to slow down as it becomes absorbed in what you are doing. There is a letting go of the day, a letting go of worries and concerns and thoughts that circle in the head. You will find that your mind becomes clear, like dirty water in a glass, once the glass is allowed to settle, the dirt goes to the bottom and the water is clear.

The normal condition of a person training in Shaolin is a tranquil, stable mind and body in balance and harmony. Shaolin helps us to find the true life force within us. The practice is very simple, just movement, breath and an open mind.

In terms of the second topic, knowing yourself, this subject is too vast for a book on kung fu so I will write about this in my third book of this series Instant Peace: Heart Advice From The Temple Of Zen.

CHAPTER FOUR

JIAN CHI - NEVER GIVE UP

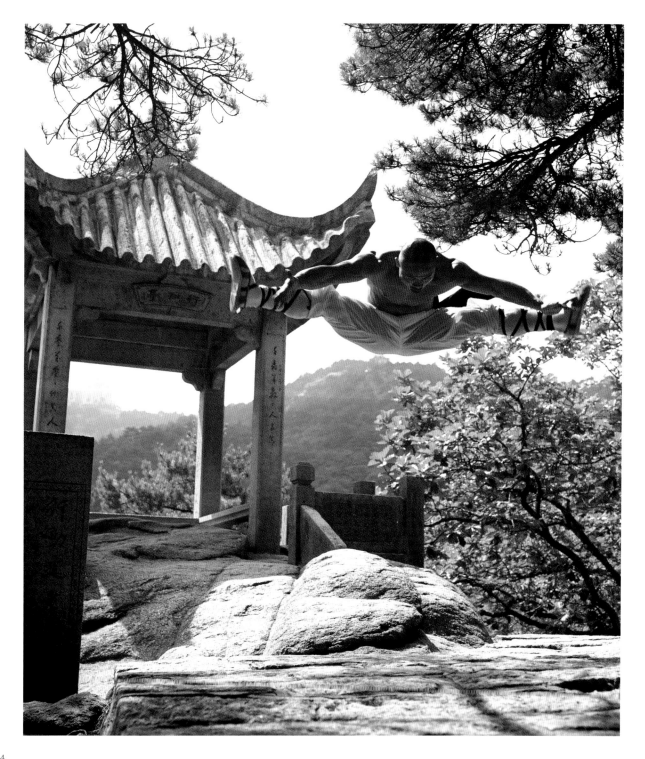

CORRECT DISCIPLINE
DISTRACTION DVD EQUIPMENT
FAMILY FLEXIBILITY FINDING
FOCUS FORM HARD INJURY
KIDS KNOWLEDGE KUNG FU
MIND LIFE LAZINESS
MOTIVATION PARTNER
QI GONG PRACTICE
SCHEDULE SPACE
STAYING TRAINING

It's important when you embark on your Shaolin Path to give yourself no choice. The first stage of the martial artist is "Jian Chi" which means Never Give Up. Once we've planted this seed in our mind then our practice is the cultivation so that we can grow into a Shaolin Warrior. Setting our motivation is important because it means we know exactly which direction we want to go to. It's a little like sitting on an aeroplane, once we've taken off, we can't change our mind and say actually I want to go to Chicago or Beijing or Munich. We are on our path and we can relax knowing that we are on course and heading in the right direction.

Before you embark on your Shaolin Warrior journey, it's good to be aware of some of the pitfalls that you can fall into.

DISTRACTION AND LAZINESS

To combat laziness think about the benefits of your training. If you're training in the morning then put your alarm clock somewhere you have to get out of bed to turn it off then don't allow the thought of getting back into bed to enter your head. Have your training clothes ready and immediately get dressed into them. Yes, you can stay in bed and sleep for another hour or watch TV for another hour but think about the cause and effect of what you do. Does watching TV take you closer to your goal of being a Shaolin Warrior?

FAMILY

You need to accept that you may not be able to train as much as you used to before you had a family and you need to find strategic ways to train such as snatching time; ten minutes here and there to do some Qigong, find ways to stretch in your daily life, for example rather than bending down to pick up a toy, keep your legs straight and stretch your muscles as you pick up the toy. Keep in mind that giving time to yourself to train adds years to your life and energy to yourself so that you can give more time and love to your family.

INJURY

Do Qigong. This will help your injury to heal. If you need to adapt the Qigong so that it doesn't aggravate your injury then go ahead and do this. When you first embark on your training you may get injured. A lot of time this is an imbalance in your body that you weren't aware of before because you never pushed your body. Once these imbalances are corrected, you shouldn't get many injuries from the training. It is safe because we don't use equipment but our own body as a weight and this lessens the likelihood of injury. Another thing you can do when your injured is go through the forms in your mind. Visualise each movement step by step as if your body is really doing the form. Don't get angry with yourself, use this time wisely, nothing is wasted.

LACK OF FOCUS

Decide what your goal is, do you want to be a martial artist? If so, why? Do you want to increase your fitness? Pinpoint the why and this will help you stay on course. Shaolin forms increase your focus through increasing your moment-to-moment awareness. Keep a note of your progression either by filming yourself or writing down details of your training sessions. What is the quality of your kick? How low is your horse stance? Has the quality of your mind changed since beginning the practice? Be realistic about what you can do and work from there.

LACK OF A PARTNER

I've formed a Facebook page for people who train with my books and DVDs, join that page to encourage each other on your Shaolin Journey. You may even be able to find someone in your area who you can link up with and start training together. I do a Shaolin Summer Camp every summer in Henan Province, China, a few kilometres away from the Shaolin Temple. Come and train in the summer and meet fellow Shaolin Warriors.

LACK OF TIME

Shaolin Martial Arts is a medicine; it prevents illness that comes through stress, lack of exercises and poor diet, so take the time now so that you can add more years to your life. Once we are ill, we have no choice but to stay in hospital or rest or lie in bed, we no longer think, I don't have the time. So give yourself no choice now.

SPACE

All of the training in this book can be done in the space the size of a yoga mat. If you have people living underneath you, then challenge yourself to train quietly when you do the forms and the kicks as they should be done lightly and not heavily. Of course, with the stamina work this isn't possible but again it's about finding creative ways around what limitations you have. There's always a way. Wherever I go, I find somewhere to train even if it's a car park. Nowhere to run? Then skip.

DISCIPLINE

Research has shown that there's a limit to will power, it's a little like petrol, after awhile it runs out, this is why we must replace will power with habit. How do we do this? I know that in the West many of you drink coffee in the morning and without your coffee you feel you can't start your day. When you were born you didn't drink coffee, it's something you started to do as adults and now your body expects it and your mind is on automatic, preparing and drinking the coffee without even thinking about it. You need to get to the same level of automation with your training and you do this through consistent regular practice on the same days and at the same time. Train at the same days and times every week. Within a few weeks, if you don't train then you will find that your body misses the training, it's expecting it, you won't be able to relax until you have done your training.

I'M TOO OLD

If you're starting your training in your forties, fifties or sixties then you won't be able to do the splits, deep stances or be a spectacular martial artist but you will be stronger, fitter, healthier, happier and have increased energy. Trying to go into the splits means you open your hips and stretch your legs at the same time so it's good to attempt it. Every summer my sister comes to help me with my Shaolin Summer Camp. She's 56 years old, has just started training now and she loves it. Why? Because she has an increase in energy, has lost weight, and feels young again. A flexible body means a flexible mind.

We can think of a thousand and one excuses not to train but they are excuses, the trick is finding creative ways around the limitations of our lives. The limitations we have in our training are limitations we have in our life so start dismantling your prison and set yourself free.

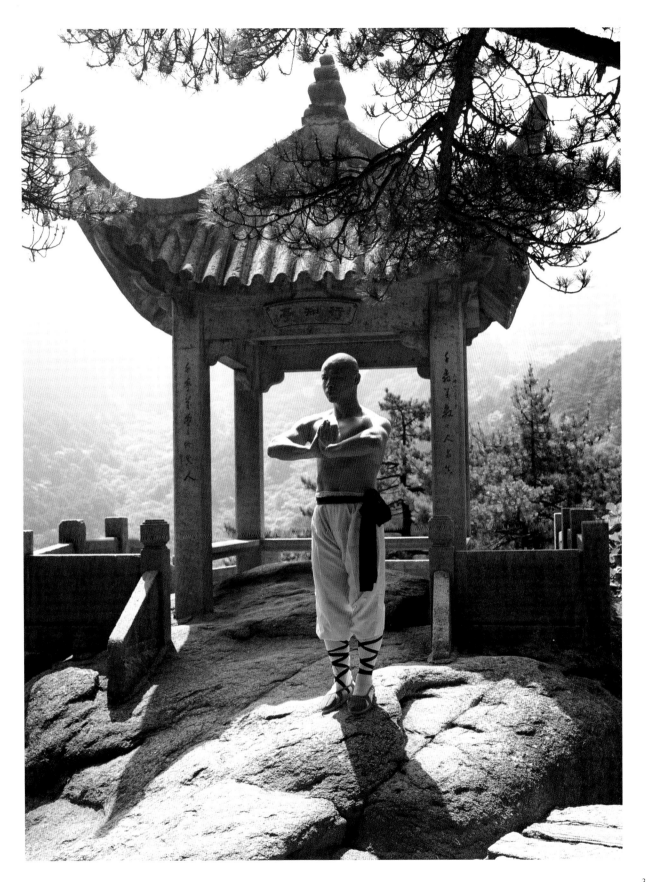

CHAPTER FIVE

MY SHAOLIN JOURNEY

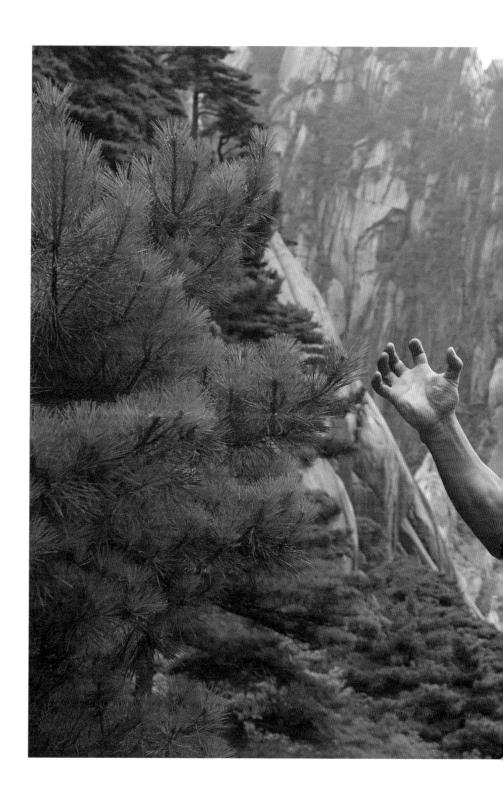

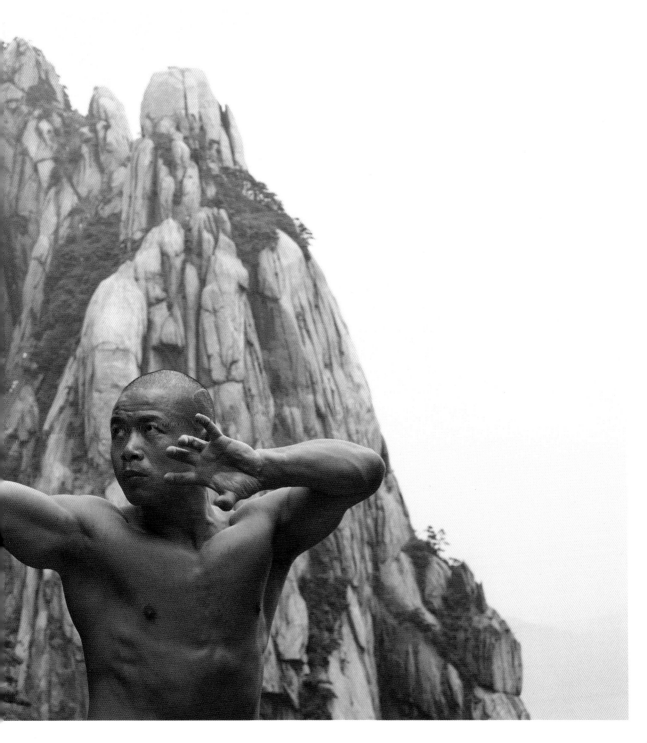

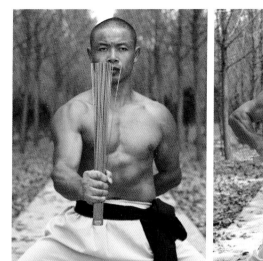
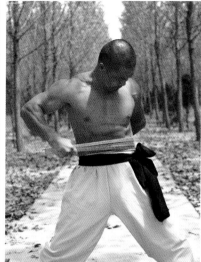
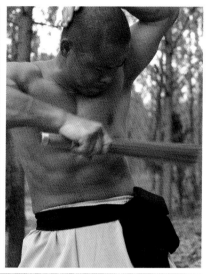
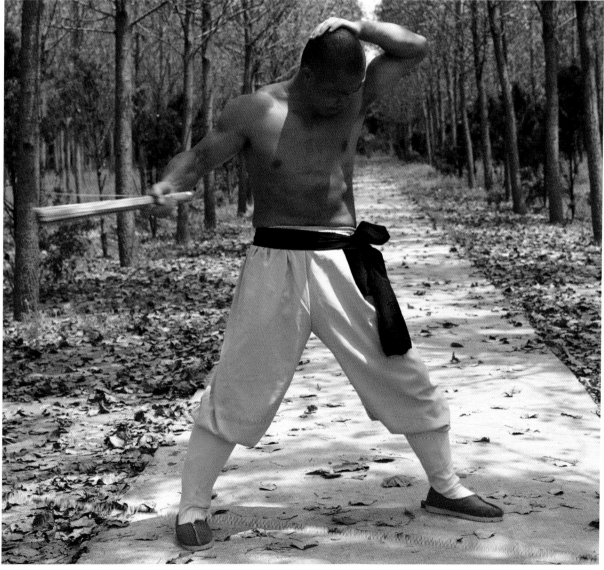

Before you begin on your journey to Shaolin, I would like to share with you a little of how I became a Shaolin Temple disciple.

I come from the largest province in China. Encircled by mountains, Xin Jiang borders on Mongolia, Russia and Pakistan. The population is a mix of Han Chinese and Muslim Uyghur and our food reflects this. We eat spicy lamb, handmade noodles and flat bread made from milk and sesame that we bake in a brick oven. I miss this food now that I live in the West.

Of course, when I was growing up I didn't have access to this abundance of food. Like most people in China, my family were so poor that my parents struggled to feed us. From December through to April our diet consisted of potatoes, carrots, onions and steamed bread. We hardly ever ate fish or meat, and as a child I was used to the constant pang of hunger.

I am the youngest of three brothers and three sisters, which meant that as the political climate began to change, I was the only one in our family who would have the opportunity to go to school and onto university. It took a lot of persuasion before my family let me study at the Shaolin Temple but I was determined.

Because I was the youngest, my brothers were always bullying me, and being the smallest boy in my year meant I also got bullied at school. My dream was to become a great fighter so I would come back to my province a hero and beat up every one that had wronged me.

When I was fourteen I knelt at my father's bed and asked him to allow me to go and train at the Shaolin Temple. When he woke up in the morning I was still there. He didn't say yes or no, but drove me to the station.

I was very excited because I had never travelled by train before. The journey took three days by train and another five hours by bus. When I got to Henan Province everything was new to me. Even the food was totally different to what I was used to. I had never seen a car before, I had never seen so many shops, and I walked around like a tourist taking everything in.

At the temple I shared a room with twenty other boys who were all about my age. At 5.30 am we were woken. We had fifteen minutes to wash and go to the toilet before we lined up at 5.45 and waited for our teacher. We then ran up the Song Shan Mountain to the Bodhidharma cave, our feet in rhythm with each other. Once we came back we began our martial training of kicks, stances, jumps, punches and forms.

We were also taught a lot of acrobatics and forms for performance and demonstration. They looked beautiful and impressive but my main motivation was to learn how to fight and this is what I focused on. I think this may be one of the reasons my master – The Shaolin Abbot Shi Yong Xin - gave me the disciple name of Lei, which means thunder.

Outside the temple I began to test the techniques I had learnt against the older boys who had been here longer than me. Sometimes I would get into such big fights that I'd be arrested and held at the local police station. My Master got tired of coming to release me so he sent me to a Ch'an Temple in another province in the hope that I would calm down.

The Abbot in this temple was a remarkable man. He was the only monk who had remained in the temple when the Red Guards had come. They had beaten him and burnt down most of the temple but still he stayed. He struggled to eat and keep warm but now Buddhism was allowed and the temple was beginning to flourish again.

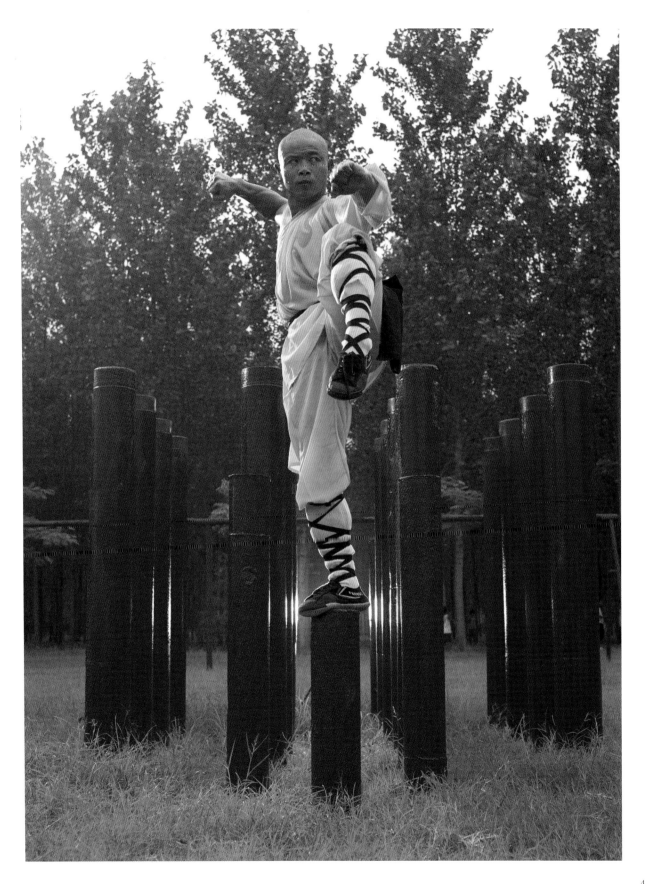

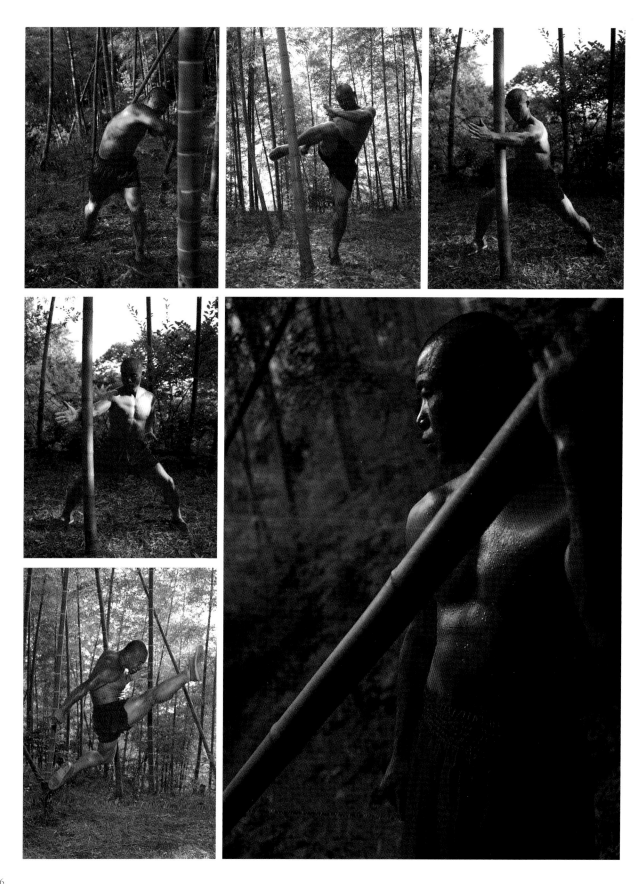

I would go with him when he gave teachings to lay people and in return for the teachings they would offer a donation to help with the cost of re-building the temple. He would wake me in the early hours of the morning and ask me to come and chant with him but I explained to him that I couldn't concentrate. So he asked me what I could concentrate on. I told him: my training. He then instructed me to let my training be my meditation. Just this one sentence changed my life and I suddenly understood why Shaolin martial arts is linked with Buddhism. Through training our body we train our mind.

From that day on, while he chanted I trained. And when I was seventeen he asked me to be ordained as a monk but I told him that I knew nothing about life so how could I become a monk?

At the Shaolin Temple, there are seventy-two different styles and when I returned to the Shaolin Temple my Master told me to specialize in one of them. I decided to choose Shaolin Steel Jacket because I wanted to challenge myself and in some ways, challenge the Shaolin teaching. I had been taught so much performance that I was confused about what was real and what wasn't, and I had to find out for myself.

When people demonstrate Shaolin Steel Jacket, they usually break sticks across their body but this is not real Shaolin Steel Jacket, it is possible to break sticks with muscle alone. Steel Jacket is a fifty - fifty combination of internal and external training, which combines Qigong exercises with intense stamina training and body conditioning. I direct my Qi into my ribs and use bricks or an iron bar to beat myself. My Qi protects my body from injury. But the highest level of Shaolin Steel Jacket is to make our body like a diamond so that disease cannot penetrate.

As I have got older, I've found another way to practise Shaolin Steel Jacket with more of a focus on health and fitness than martial power. I'm still interested in fighting and I coach fighters because I believe it's good for a young person to be challenged in the ring; many young people seem lost and the discipline can give direction to their life and help them to contribute more fully in our society. But I also focus on what is useful for health and fitness. What is the quickest way to instant health and fitness?

The reason I ask that question is because I don't want to waste my time or my student's time. I want to teach them skills that are useful for their life, whether that is fighting stress and fitness levels or fighting an opponent in the ring. Both of these are challenges and we need to cultivate the energy of a warrior to succeed.

After I left the temple, I travelled to other martial arts schools both to learn from different masters and teach what I had learnt at the Temple. In 2000, I was asked by my brother Shifu Shi Yan Zi to come to London and help set up the first Shaolin Temple in Europe. The Abbot was concerned about the spread of un-authentic Shaolin teachings so he wanted a Shaolin Temple in the UK. Up until that time, Shifu Yan Zi and I had only taught students who trained full-time, so we had to find a way to condense the teachings into two hours.

Seeing that Shaolin was having a positive effect on our students which went way beyond the health benefits, I went on to make a series of Shaolin Warrior DVDs so I could share with as many people as possible the true teachings from the Shaolin Temple. I then wrote my first book, Instant Health: The Shaolin Qigong Workout For Longevity, which is now in its third publication.

When you step onto the path of Shaolin, you are taking on a tradition which is thousands of years old. Shaolin contains The Tao, Confucius and Zen Buddhism; this is why I decided to shoot the photographs in this book in China. I wanted to return to the roots of martial arts and demonstrate the origins of the teachings. They come from the mountains, the bamboo forests, the rice fields and the traditional villages of China. It is this landscape that has given the forms their shape.

Today the majority of us practise in an urban environment. Many of my students are now based in London, New York, Paris and Beijing. As China as has prospered, so have they. When my Chinese students came to visit me at the temple, they thanked me for teaching them Shaolin as it has given them the determination, confidence and willpower to succeed as successful businessmen.

I am not a great martial artist which is why I'm always training and always learning. I am not the greatest teacher but I try to give a taste of what Shaolin really is. It's not a dream or a fantasy like it is sometimes made out to be, but the art and science of true health and happiness.

I believe there are no bad students: there are just bad teachers, and if you choose to study from my books then you become my student and I hope I will teach you well.

As you can see from my story I am not a perfect person. The Buddha's flower is the lotus and it grows from mud. Whatever place you are in right now, whatever problems or difficulties you may have, you can use these problems to grow something beautiful through the guidance of the Shaolin teachings.

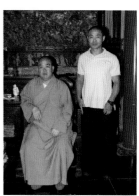

Yan Lei with his master
The Shaolin Abbot Shi Youg Xiu

PART TWO

THE FUNDAMENTAL OF SHAOLIN KUNG FU

CHAPTER SIX
KUNG FU BREATHING

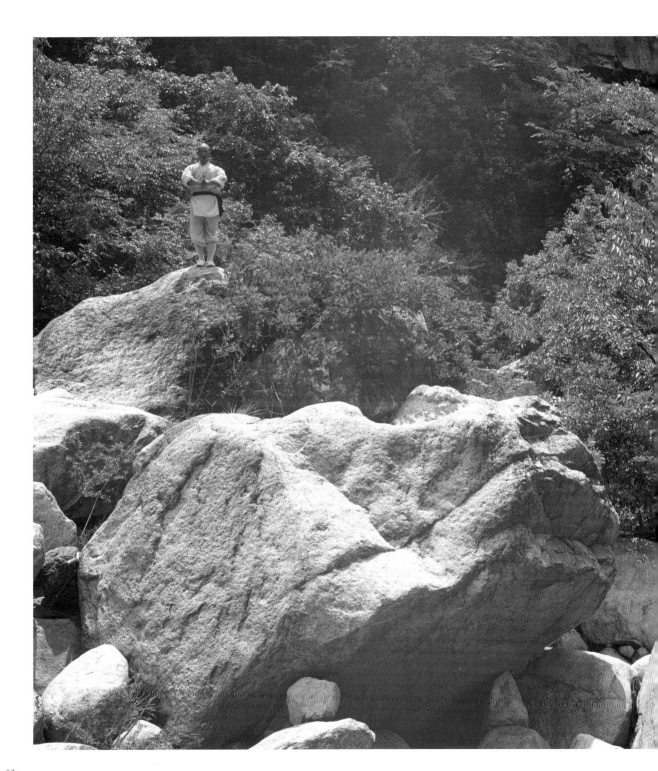

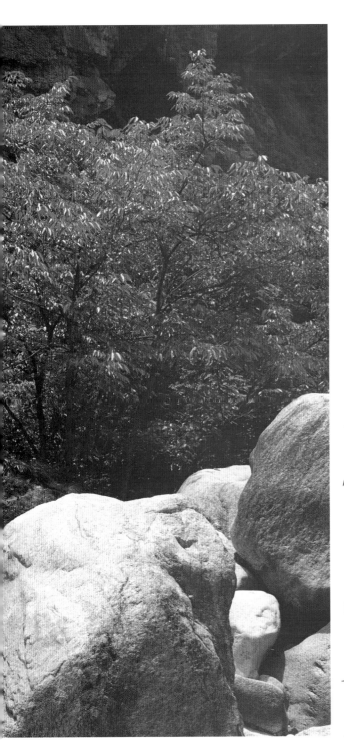

BREATH IS
THE LINK
BETWEEN
OUR BODY
AND OUR
MIND.

There is a famous Zen story about a disciple who was told to meditate on the breath. After a few months, the disciple said to his master that he found breathing boring. The master took hold of the disciple's head and held it down in a bucket of water. "Now do you find breathing boring?"

Breath is the link between our body and our mind. It's a barometer of our feelings. When we feel anxious, our breathing quickens, when we feel peaceful, our breathing slows down.

When you do the warm up, stamina training and stretching, use normal abdominal breathing. When you practice kung fu, you need to breathe in the same way as when you practice Qigong. When you inhale, your stomach goes in, and when you exhale, your stomach goes out. This is called reverse breathing because your stomach does the reverse of what it does when you breathe in your day-to-day life.

If you've never done this breathing before then begin by placing your left hand on your side, just below your chest and your right hand on your abdomen. Inhale - your diaphragm will contract and your abdomen will contract, at the same time your chest will expand. Exhale - your diaphragm and stomach will expand. Make sure your shoulders don't rise and fall and that you're not just breathing shallowly into your chest. If you're practicing correctly you will feel an expansion in the lungs and your breath will naturally deepen and lengthen.

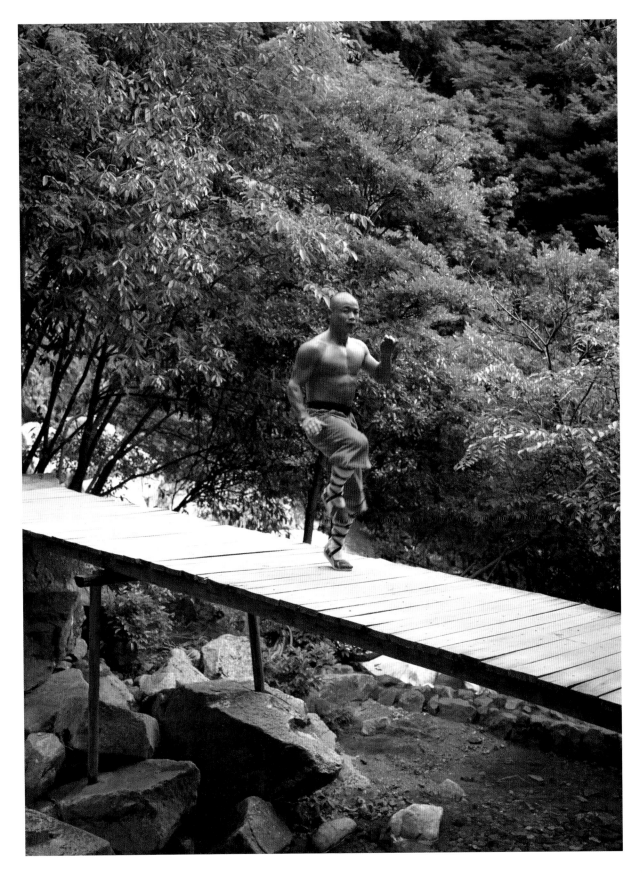

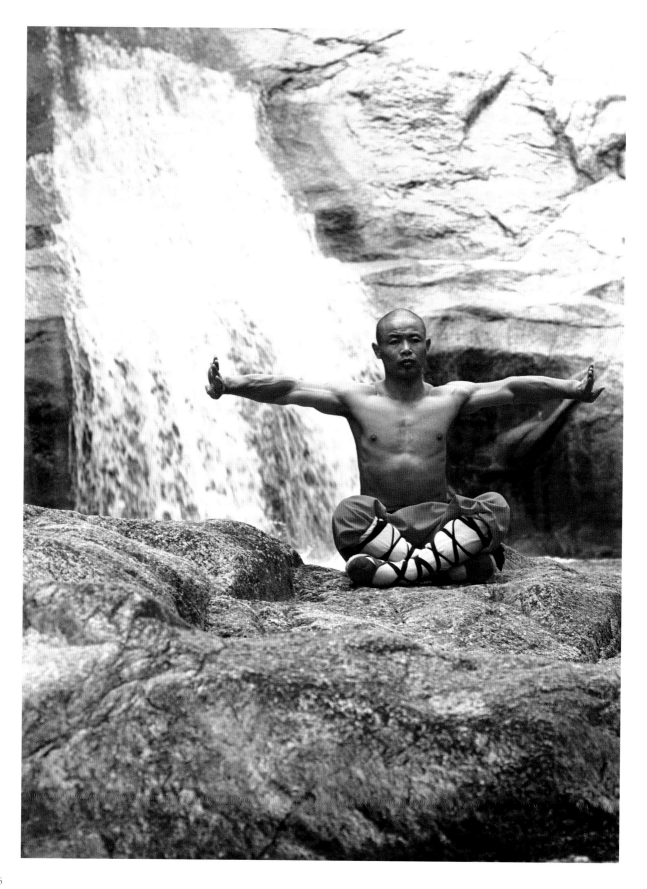

Although this method of breathing will feel strange at first, it is important to get it right. Once you have mastered the breathing, you can then pull in the perineum on the inhale and when you exhale relax the perineum. Don't pull it in 100 % as this creates tension in the body, just pull in a little. If you are a total beginner then you don't need to do this until you have fully mastered the breathing and the movement. Correct breathing gives power to your movement. It increases the length of time you can train. In order to have power, you need to be in control of your breathing.

In Kung Fu, you breathe in through the nose and out through the mouth. Often the in breath is quick and sharp, for example when you prepare at the beginning of a form or for the Five Fundamental Kicks, as you bring your clenched fists to your waist, inhale through your nose quickly and with power. The breathing is audible. In Qigong, once you have mastered the form; your breathing becomes almost inaudible. Every kick or punch you do is done on the out breath. Sometimes the in breath is held as you move into a movement then on the punch, you breathe out. You don't breathe out on the preparation of the punch.

If you're feeling confused about the breathing it means you're thinking too much. Take a simple push up, all you have to do is find the preparation or start point. This shows you where the inhale is. It's a little like diving into water. You don't exhale to prepare then dive in as you inhale. It feels very unnatural to punch or kick on an inhale. Our body knows when it needs to breathe.

As you move through the forms be aware of the rhythm of your breath, it changes as the movement changes. When you sit, your breathing is regular, the inhale and exhale happen at about the same time. But when you do a form, the inhale and exhale are dependent on the movement, they work with the movement, they change rhythm and texture; sometimes the breath is sharp and quick, sometimes it is held, sometimes it is forceful. Never forget the breath. But at the same time it mustn't be forced or laboured. There should be a naturalness and flow to it. Allow the intelligence of the Shaolin practice to take over your body. As you leave your mind behind, your breath will breathe by itself.

CHAPTER SEVEN

POSTURE AND MIND

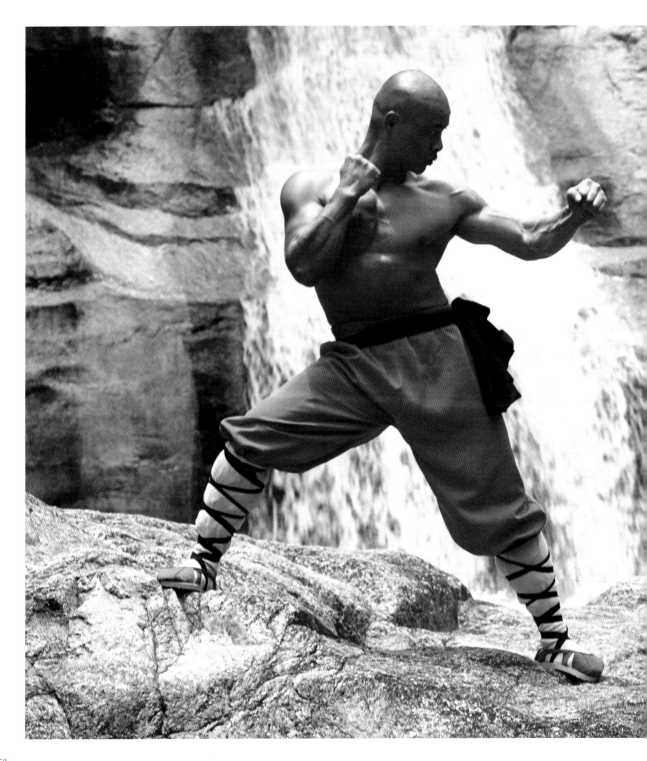

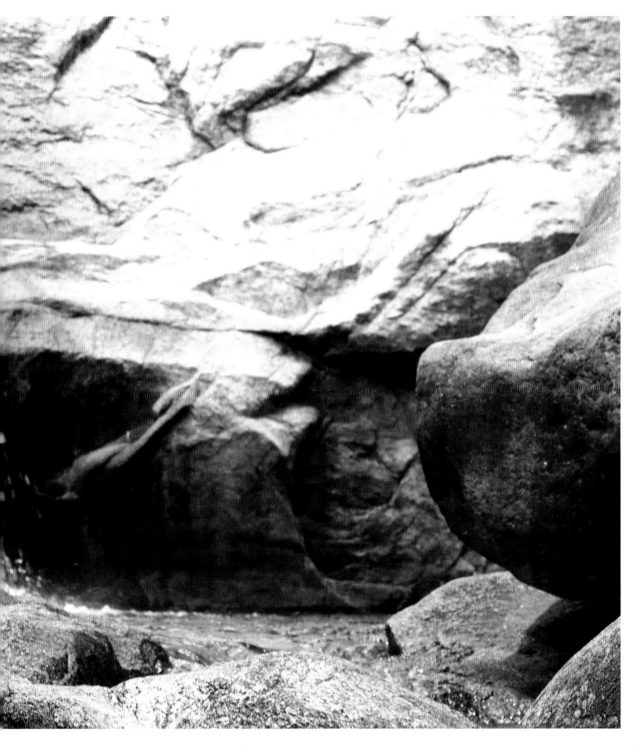

POSTURE

The body is relaxed but not lazy, straight but not stiff. If the spine is bent or crooked then the Qi cannot flow properly.

To lengthen the spine, imagine that your head is suspended from above as though a string were attached to the crown, roll your hips slightly forward so there is a gentle tucking in of the pelvis. Open your chest a little and keep your shoulders down and relaxed. Check that your knees are straight but not locked. Feel the weight of your body evenly on both feet.

Think of a tree — a tree is not tense but is stable and grounded.

Whether we do Qigong or Kung Fu, our feet always grab the floor but they do so in a natural way. At first it will feel tense and unnatural but over time your body will find a relaxed way of doing this. The state of our posture has a surprising effect on our mind. Simply standing straight can help to increase positive feelings.

MIND

It is important that when we begin our training, we focus completely on what we are doing and let go of any worries or concerns we may have. Worries circle in our mind, and the more we think, the more momentum our worries gain. The Shaolin Kung Fu Workout acts as a pair of scissors, cutting through our thoughts and giving our mind and body a place of refuge and stillness.

There is a famous story about one of Buddha's disciples called Shravana. He was a very good guitar player but was having trouble meditating, so he went to the Buddha to ask for advice. The Buddha asked Shravana,

'Does the sound of the guitar come from tight strings or loose strings?' Shravana replied, 'Neither, it is produced by balancing the strings.' The Buddha said, 'It is the same with the mind. The way to meditate is by being tight and relaxed."

And this holds true for your Kung Fu Workout. It is important to approach your training with the right attitude so that your mind is working with your body rather than opposing it. As beginners, we tend to be more tight than relaxed but over time we learn the correct way to practise. Say to yourself, you already are what you want to become.

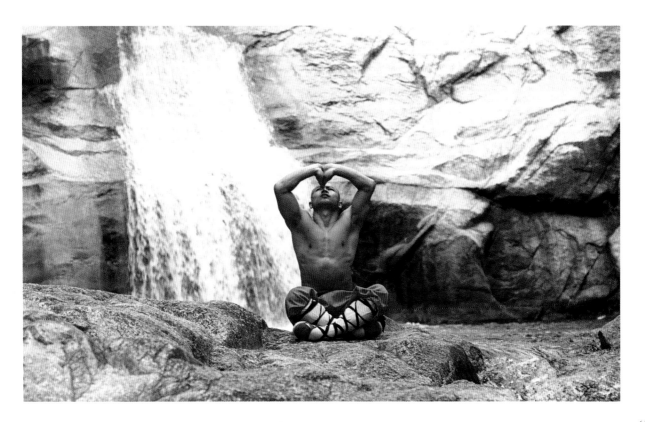

CHAPTER EIGHT

LIVING THE LIFE OF A SHAOLIN WARRIOR

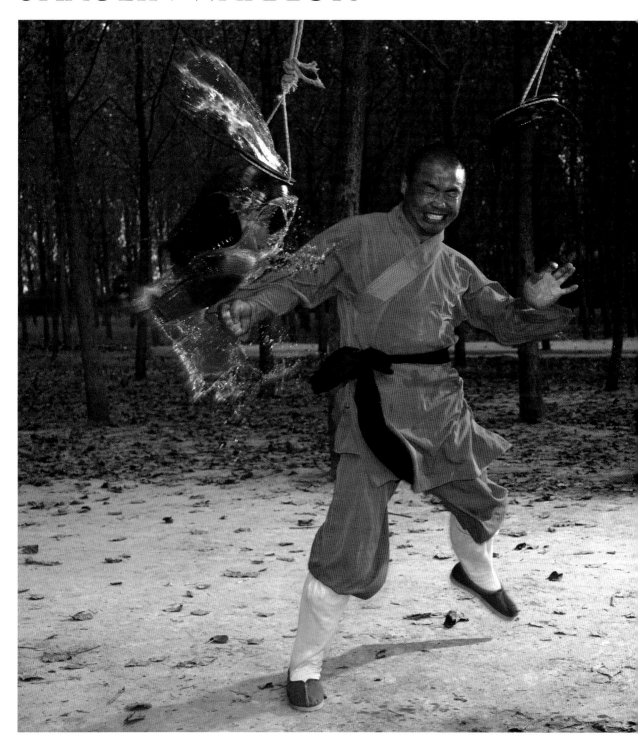

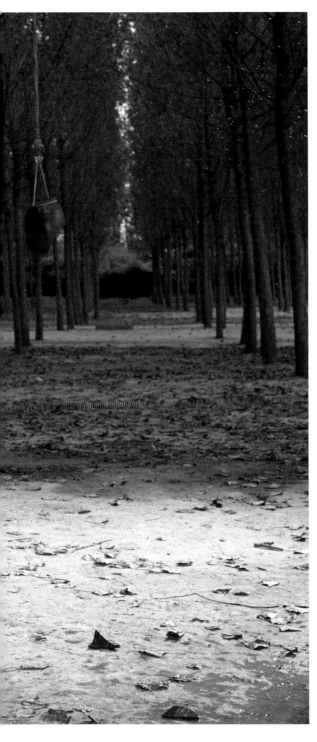

I WANT TO
INSPIRE
PEOPLE TO BE
THEIR BEST
AND REACH
THEIR FULL
POTENTIAL AS
A PERSON.

Even though I no longer live at the Shaolin Temple, my life is still very similar; I get up early, eat breakfast and train. I don't have too many desires or things as this would distract me from my goal to be the best martial artist I can be. I want to inspire people to be their best and reach their full potential as a person. I want to help people stay on the healthy path.

Sometimes I get emails from students who say they want to give up their Western life or they want to come to China and train full time. You can still be in the West and give up the things that you find negative about Western life. You don't need to come to China to train in Shaolin. If you want to be a vegetarian then be a vegetarian, it doesn't mean that the supermarket should no longer stock meat.

It's about being realistic and understanding the difference between dream and reality. Dreams are distractions. If we want something, we must work with what we have to get it and not believe it's in another country or that someone can give us that thing that we need. It's about taking responsibility and making the right choices.

In order to gain things we have to give up things. We can't have a busy social life and be a great martial artist. We can't drink a lot of alcohol and expect to be a great martial artist, drinking occasionally is okay but not on a regular basis. We can't smoke. I refuse to teach anyone who smokes. Smoking doesn't make sense if you are a martial artist. It goes against everything that we cultivate. And it's the same with drugs. This isn't about being moralistic. Alcohol and drugs muddy the mind. What we are cultivating is a clear mind.

A farmer plants seeds, but this is not enough, she also has to give it the right conditions in order for it to grow. We are no different. We all have the potential to be a Shaolin Warrior, if we give our mind and body the right conditions, then, without a doubt, we will grow into a Shaolin Warrior. This means eating well. Sleeping well. Having a simple focused life. Not too complicated. Not too many desires. And most importantly putting the action in.

When I was seven years old, my mother asked me if I had dream? I said, "Yes, I want to become a martial artist." She then asked me, "Do you know which is the highest part of your body?" I said, "My head and my hair." My mum said, "No, it's your hands." She told me, "Your mind makes your dream happen but your mind cannot make your dream come true, only your hands can do that. This means, you can't just think, you need to do."

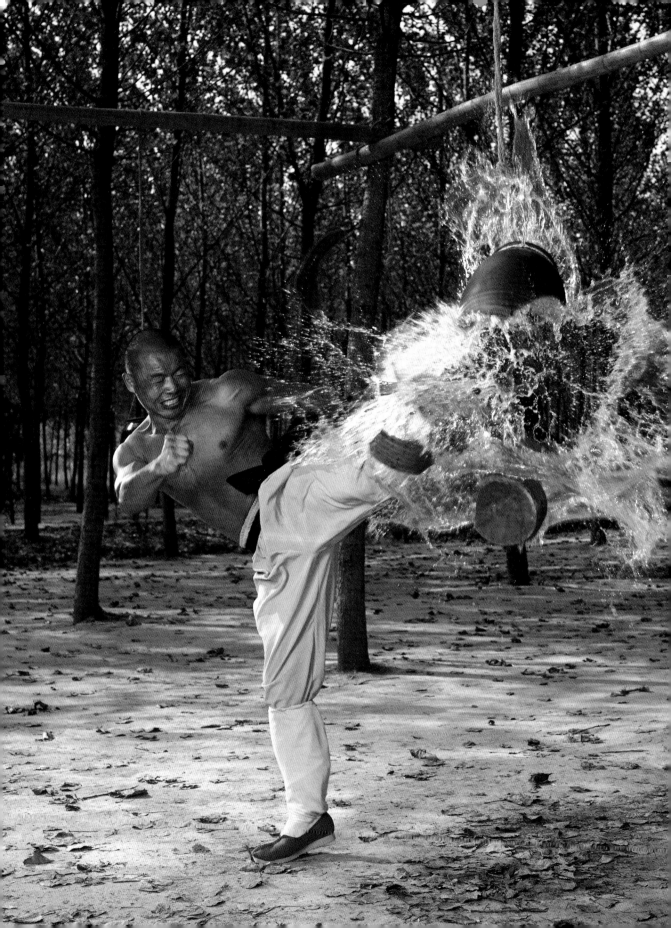

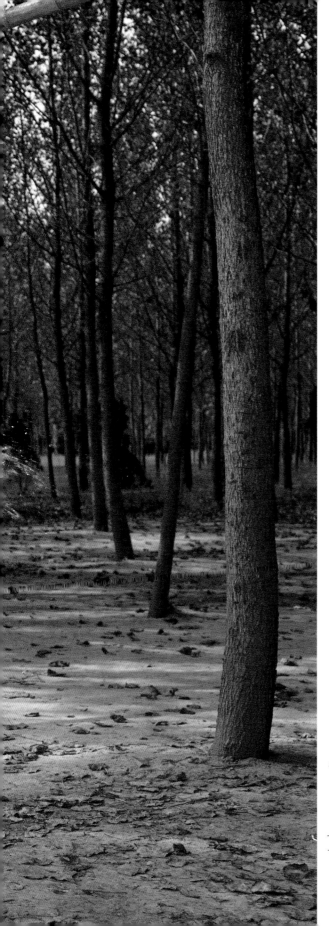

LIFE IS ABOUT
DOING, NOT
THINKING.
ACTION NOT
WORDS.

CHAPTER NINE

THE SHAOLIN WARRIOR'S DIET

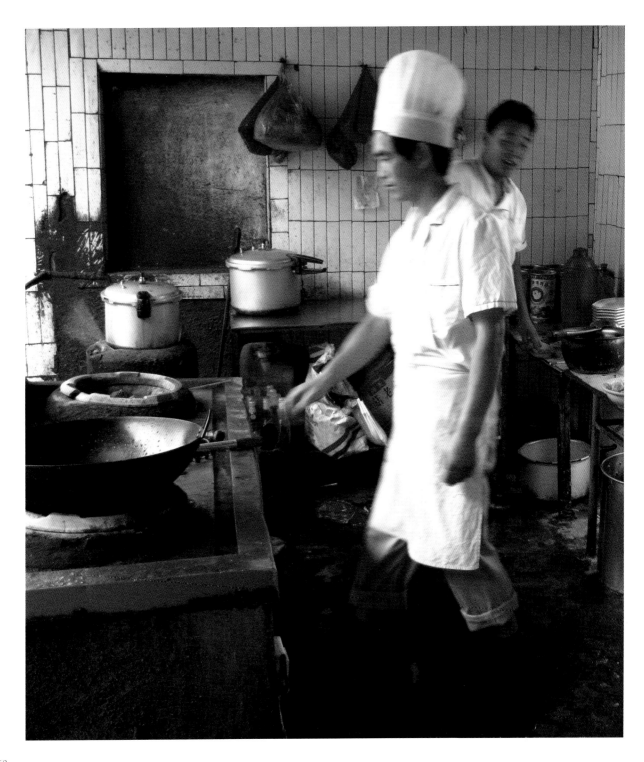

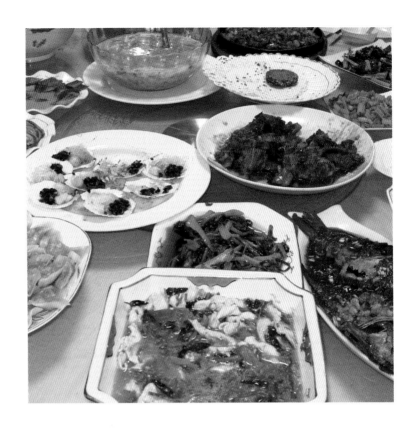

SHAOLIN MONKS, ALONGSIDE THE MAJORITY OF CHINESE PEOPLE, SEE FOOD AS MEDICINE AND EAT IN ACCORDANCE WITH ITS HEALTH PROPERTIES.

It's part of traditional Chinese Medicine, which is passed down to us by our parents so it's not something we study, we just know. We see foods as cold or hot and will alter what we eat in accordance with how our health is that day. For example, if we have a cold then we'll make chicken soup with dried red plums, Goji berries and ginger, an excellent tonic soup.

Inside the Shaolin Temple we eat vegetarian food but outside of the temple, the fighting monks can eat meat if they feel they need to. In this article I'm not going into the pros and cons of being a vegetarian, which is an emotive subject, but I'm going to give you an insight into our daily diet.

Shaolin Monk's focus on eating foods in their natural state. We don't eat energy bars or cereal, we don't drink coca cola, protein shakes, alcohol, or water with ice. We eat a diet which is rich in fruit, vegetables, and good quality protein. For carbohydrate we eat white rice, steamed buns or noodles. We drink water at room temperature, and green tea, which is rich in anti oxidants. For snacks we eat nuts and fruits.

Before I came to the West I'd never seen brown rice before. I, along with the majority of Chinese people don't like the taste of it so it's not something we eat. There seems to be a backlash against refined carbohydrates or even carbohydrates in general in the West. But anyone who trains hard needs to eat carbohydrates. White rice is a source of dietary fibre, which is important for a healthy digestive system; it contains vitamin B1 and is low in fat.

Our daily food is stir-fried vegetables and protein, the most common protein being lamb, chicken, pork or tofu. Lamb is usually grass fed which is better than grain fed, it's very Yang and warm and is good to eat if people are low in energy. We rarely eat beef. We eat protein with every meal because it helps us to sustain energy during our training. For our evening meal we don't eat any carbohydrate unless we're going to train that evening.

Shaolin Monks believe that the time they eat their food is as important as what they eat. We eat our heaviest food at breakfast because we need this energy for training, a slightly lighter lunch then less food in the evening.

Chinese food - excluding Chinese food in Western restaurants which is usually not authentic Chinese - combines food in such a way that not only is it packed with nutrition but it's also an immune booster.

A good dish to eat in the evening is five vegetable stir-fry with ginger. Take five vegetables, preferably five different colours, cut them thinly then stir-fry them with ginger, garlic and chilli. I suggest that one of your vegetables is red pepper, which has a high vitamin C content, and shitake mushroom, which enhances immunity. Ginger aids digestion, chilli contains capsicum which has anti-bacterial qualities and garlic is one of the most powerful healing foods that you can include in your daily diet to boost immunity. This simple dish not only tastes great but helps to prevent cancer, the common cold, gives you your five a day, and cannot make you fat.

When we eat we do eating meditation. This slows down our eating and means that we never eat too much as our digestion has time to tell us that we're full.

PART THREE
THE SHAOLIN KUNG FU WORKOUT

CHAPTER TEN

WARM UP

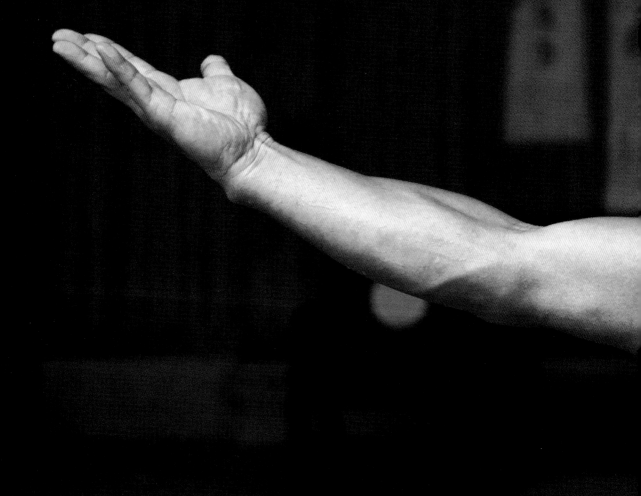

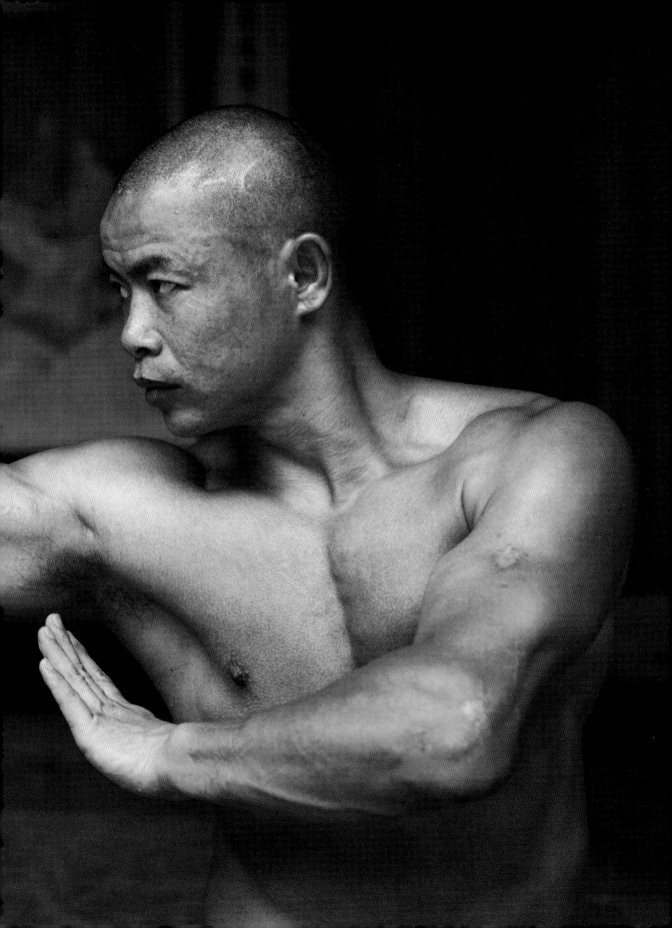

These exercises are not things we learn or do, they are what we are. Try to let go of impatience and wanting to achieve anything, and use the time you do these exercises as time out from the pressure of modern day living and a time to give something back to yourself.

There should be no pain when you do any of these exercises. If there is then stop immediately because you are either doing something incorrectly or you have an injury which means these exercises are not correct for you at this time. Take it gently; don't push yourself, especially in the morning when your muscles and joints will be at their stiffest. Listen to your body and gently build up your flexibility. It is important to do the movements correctly and not force any movements.

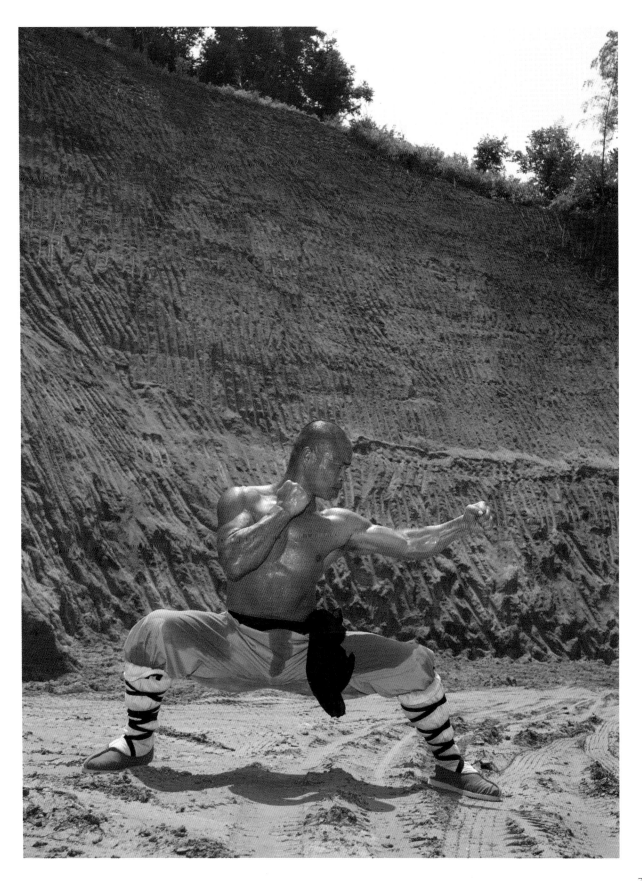

WARM UP

If we are about to embark on a long motorway journey, we usually check our car to make sure there's enough air in the tyres, and oil and water for the engine to run smoothly. At the Shaolin Temple, we check that our joints are okay before we begin our training. The warm up helps to protect us from injury and it is also a time when we can tune into our body and see which parts of the body feel stiff, tense or less flexible.

When we start to warm up, we take it slowly and focus on the part of the body that we are warming up. The warm up exercises usually take between four to seven minutes. Younger people can warm up in four minutes but if you are older, stiffer or haven't done any exercise in a while, you will need to take the full seven minutes.

LABEI
BACK STRETCH

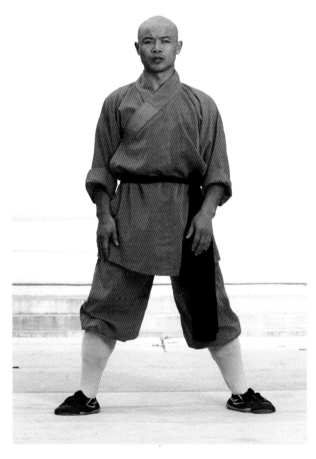

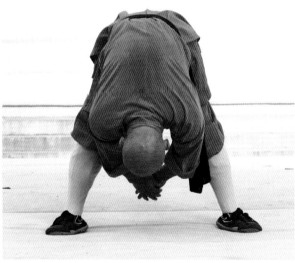

1) Open your feet hip width apart.

2) Drop your head onto your chest and fold forward vertebra by vertebra. Stretch down to the middle of your body and place your left hand over your right hand.
Very gently bounce three times in the centre then the left and the right.
REPS: 3 TO THE CENTRE AND EACH SIDE.
Make sure the knees stay straight and the neck and shoulders dropped and relaxed. The head should be like a rag doll. Check for any tension in the jaw. From this movement go straight into:

SHUAN YAO
WAIST CIRCLE

The aim is to make a complete circle with your upper body. This can be done at a speed which feels right for your body. When we are warming up for Qigong we do this exercise slowly but when we are warming up for Kung Fu we speed this movement up.

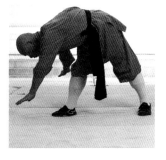 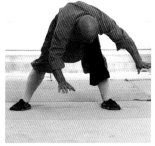

1) – 6) Open your arms and circle your body from the right to the left, continue to circle your body up to the upper left, the centre of the back, the upper right and then down to the lower right.
REPS: 3 CLOCKWISE AND 3 ANTI-CLOCKWISE.
Your eyes always follow your arms. When you fold forward, you can bend the knees a little, when you stretch up and back, straighten your legs and feel a stretch in your back.

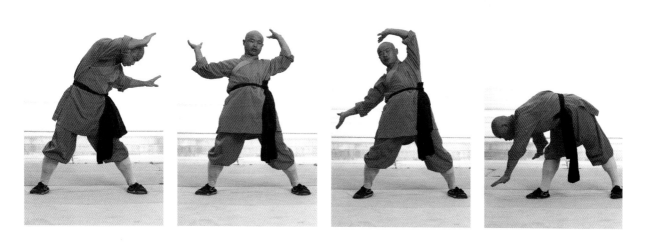

GONG BU LA JIAN
SHOULDER STRETCH
HORSE STANCE

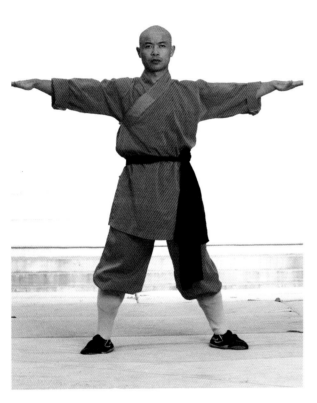

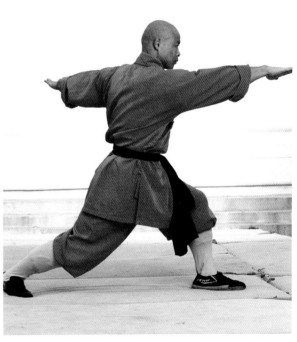

1) Open your feet slightly wider than your hips and take both arms out to the side. Keep your arms straight.

2) Turn to the left and bend your left knee slightly. Keeping your right leg straight, stretch your right arm in front of and your left arm behind you.

3) Stretch your arm forward four times then turn to the other side and repeat.
REPS: 3 EACH SIDE.

Feel a stretch in your shoulder and keep your arms as straight as possible.

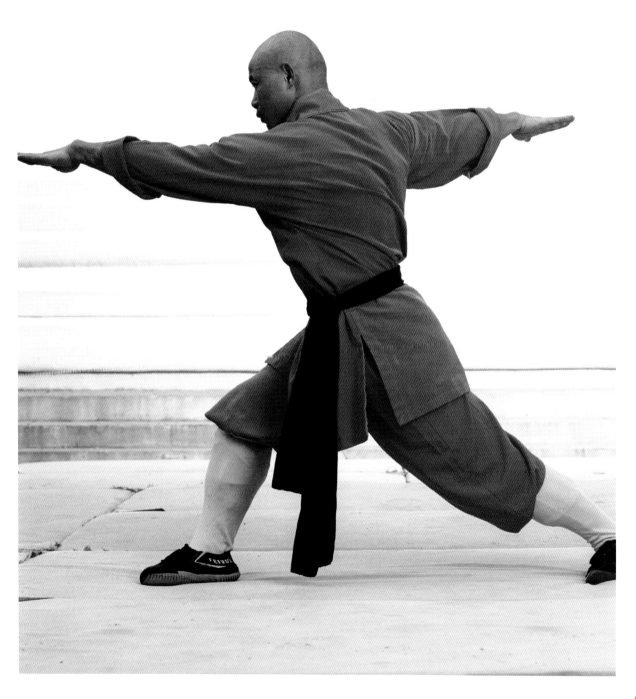

QIAN HOU FU YAO
WAIST WARM UP

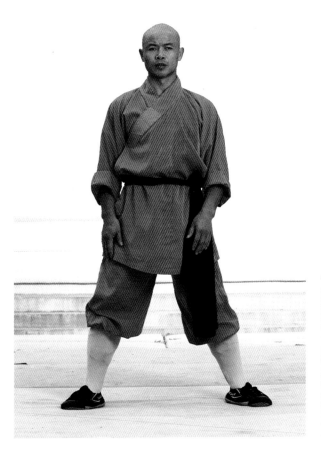

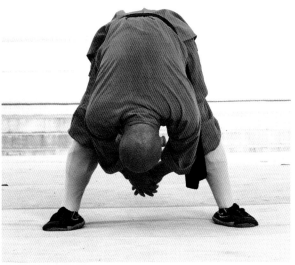

1) Open your feet hip width apart and bring your arms over your head. Place your left hand over the right hand.

2) Bend your waist and place your hands as far as possible through your legs. Inhale and exhale 3 times to lengthen the stretch.

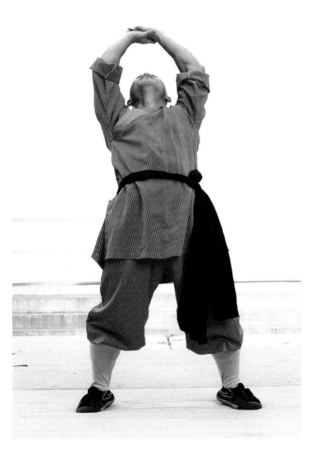

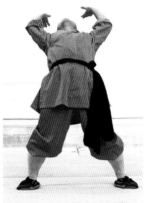

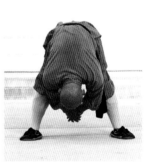

5) Bend at your waist and repeat this sequence three times.
REPS: 3
With the following exercises the emphasis is on making a circle with each of your body parts that you warm up.

3) - 4) Bring your torso upright, bend your legs slightly and stretch your back until your eyes look at the wall behind you.

NECK CIRCLE

With the following exercises the empahsis is on making a circle with each of your body parts that you warm up.

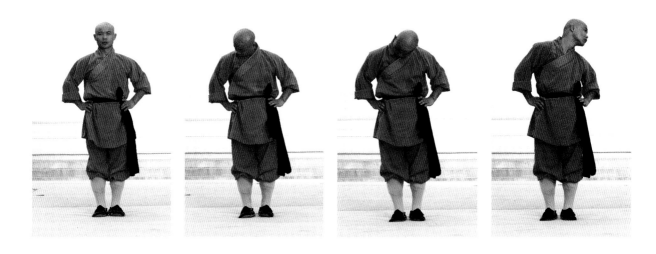

1) – 5) Close your feet, close your teeth, drop your shoulders and slowly circle your neck to the left. Let it follow your natural range of movement, inhaling as you begin moving from the back and to the right. REPS: 3 EACH DIRECTION.

Make sure you are only moving the neck for this exercise and not your shoulders or your upper body.

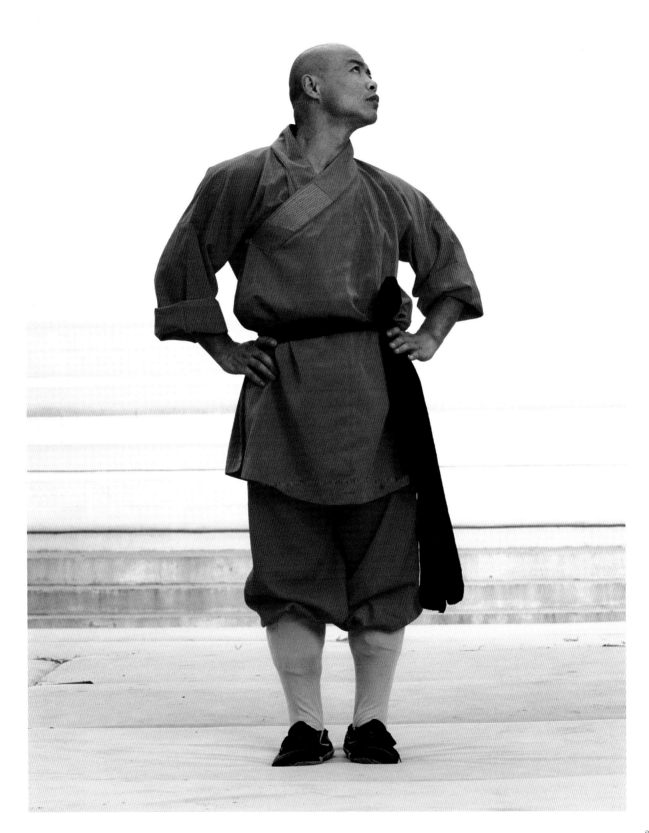

SHOULDER CIRCLE

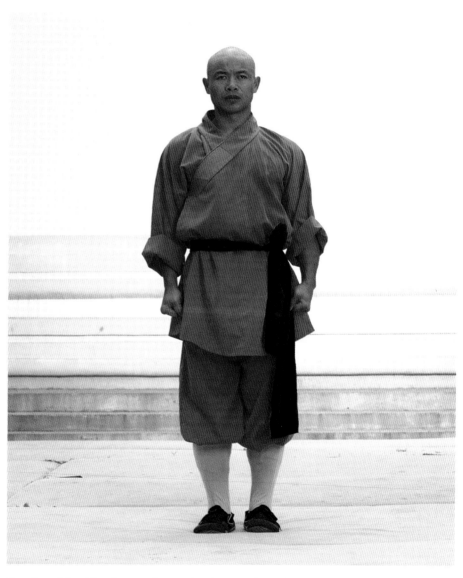

Stand straight. Clench your fists and make a circle with your shoulders in a clockwise direction.
REPEAT 3 TIMES.

2) Change sides and circle your shoulders in an anti-clockwise direction.
REPEAT 3 TIMES.

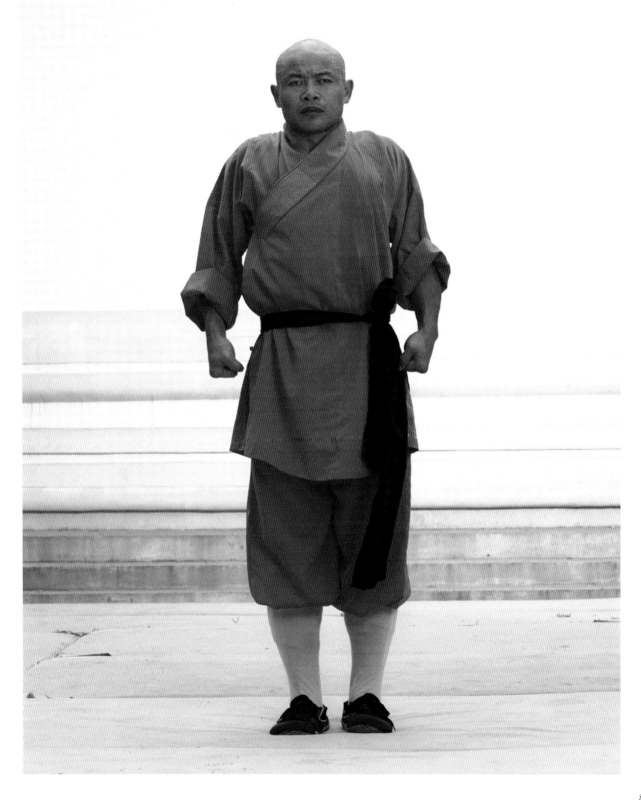

ELBOW CIRCLE

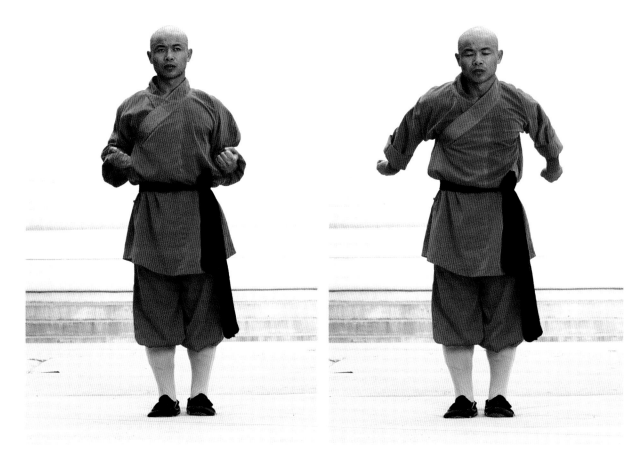

1) Clench your fists. Bend your elbows and draw your fists to your waist until your elbows can't go back anymore. Feel your chest open.

2) Turn your fists into your body and stretch your arms behind your back – feel a stretch in your arm.

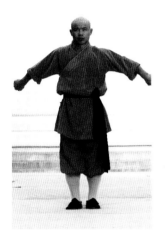 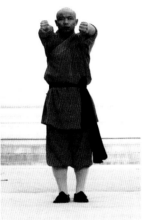 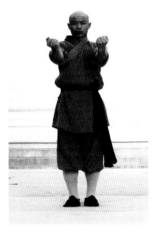

3) 4) Keep your arm straight and circle your arms to the side and then the front of your body – your knuckles should be facing inwards.

5) Turn your fists so your knuckles are facing the ground.

6) Bring your fists back to your waist.
REPS: 3

WRIST CIRCLE

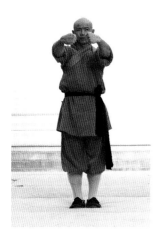 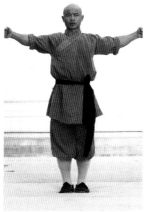 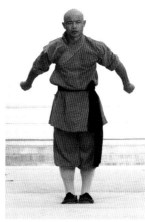 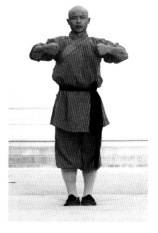

1) Clench your fists and stretch both arms straight out in front of you with the elbows pointing outwards. Bend your fists inwards until you feel a stretch in the wrist.

2) Take both arms out to the side so your shoulders and arms are in one line and your chest feels expanded.

3) Keep moving your arms until they are behind your body. When they can't go back any further…

4) 5) Bring your fists to your chest then push your fists straight out in front of you.

REPS: 3
The focus is on turning your wrist and feeling a stretch in your wrist.

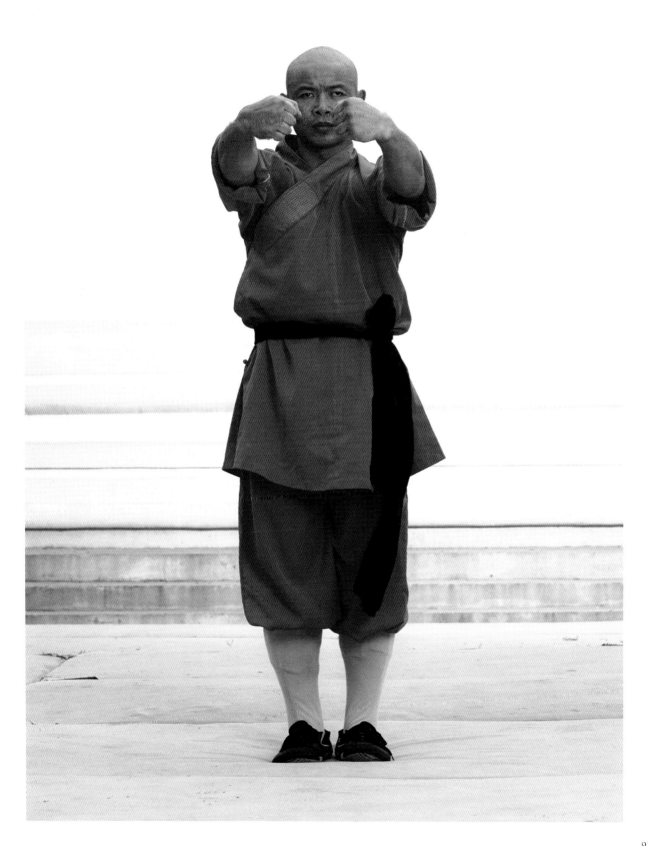

KNEE CIRCLE

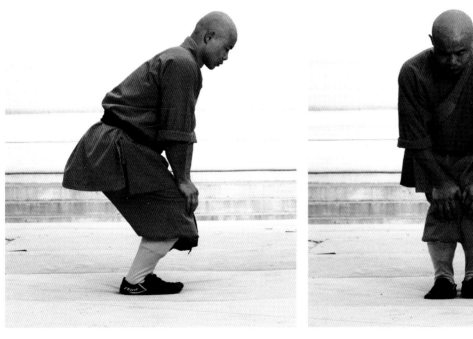
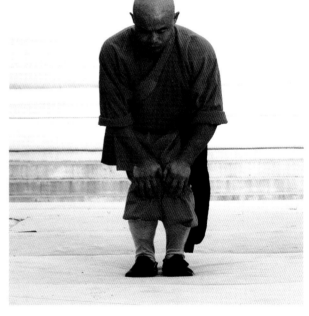

1) – 2) Bend your knees making sure to keep your back straight. Place your hands on your knees and move your knees in a circle from left to right then change direction. REPS: 3 IN EACH DIRECTION.

ANKLE CIRCLE

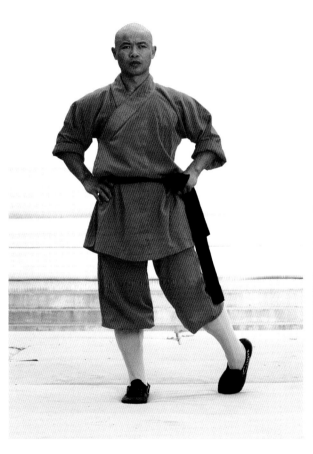

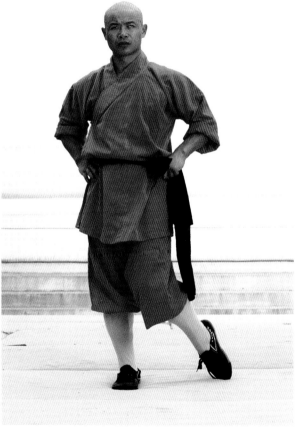

1) Balance on one leg, circle your left ankle in a clockwise direction three times. Then reverse the direction and circle the ankle counter-clockwise three times.

2) Bend your foot backwards and stretch your foot three times. Change sides and repeat.

CHAPTER ELEVEN

SHAOLIN STAMINA TRAINING

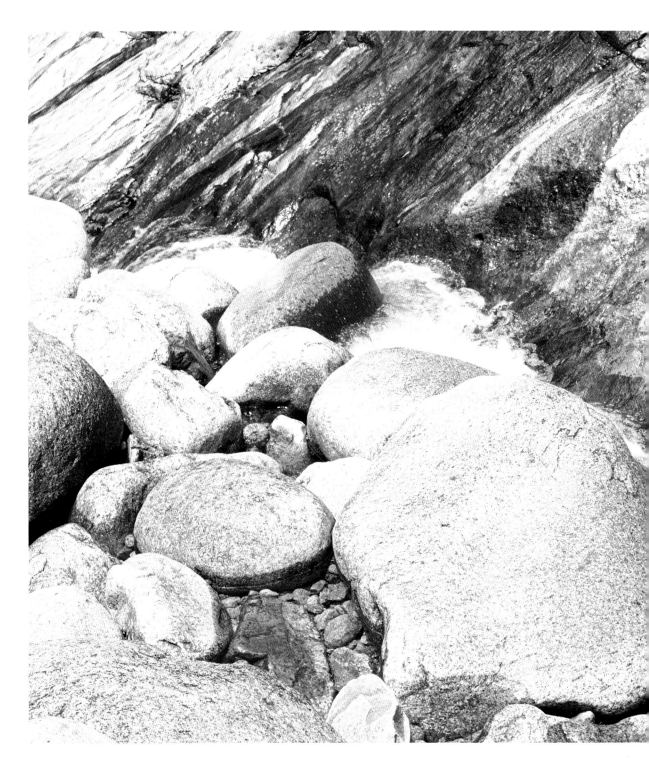

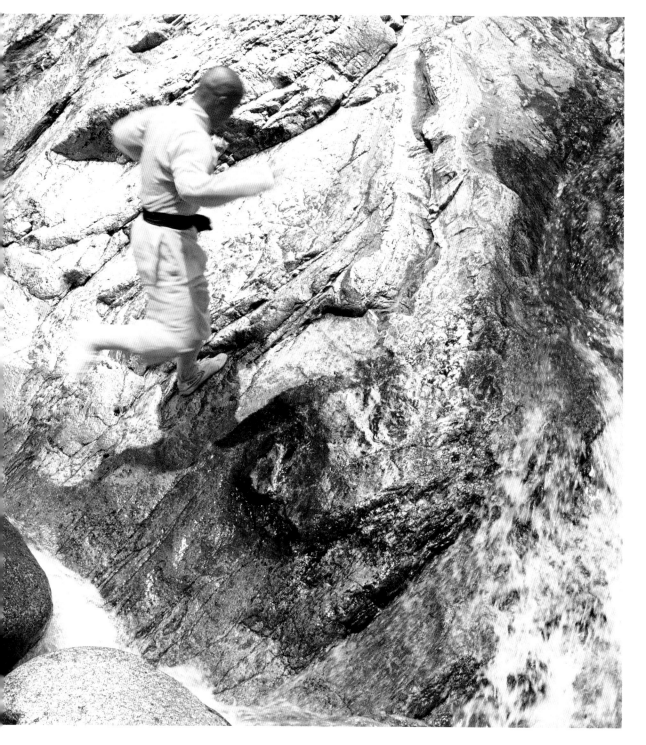

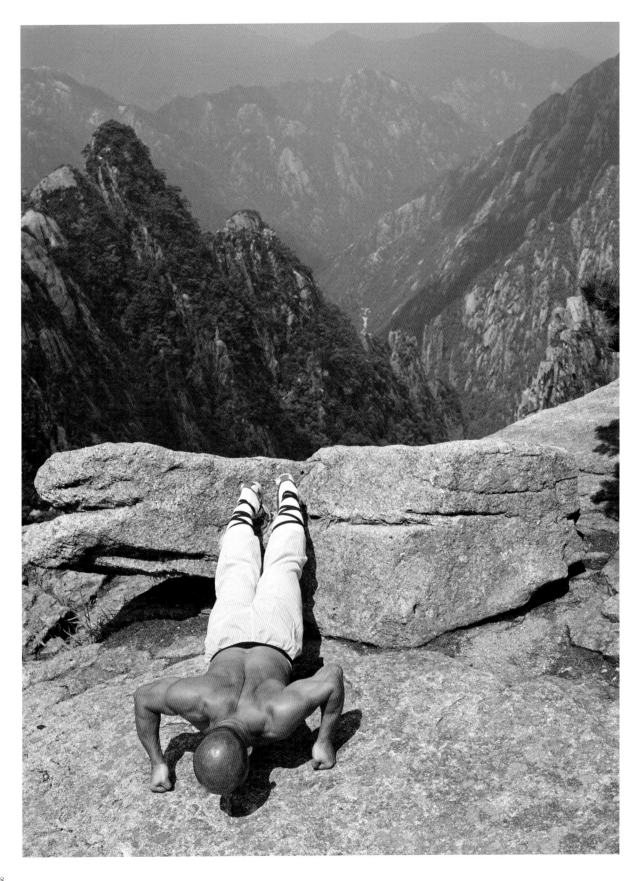

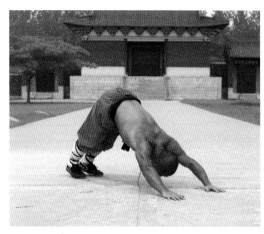

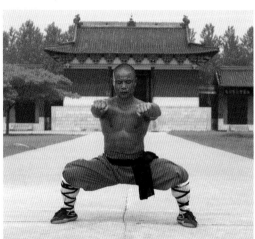

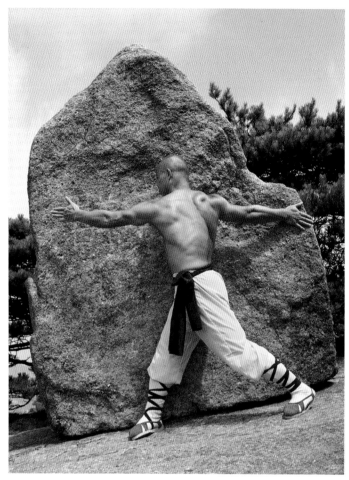

Shaolin Stamina Training consists of five simple basic exercises and yet it will challenge you whatever level you are. These five exercises work all of the major muscle groups. If you are a beginner you can leave out the Qigong press up and add it in when you are fitter.

Do three rounds of each exercise.

PUSH UP

The humble push up is an excellent exercise to strengthen the upper body. Start off by using your hands then as your body gets stronger progress onto your fists. Make sure that your back is straight and your stomach is held in. When you lower your body onto the ground, don't collapse your body onto the ground. If you have never done press-ups before then modify this by keeping your legs on the floor and pushing up your lower body rather than your whole body.

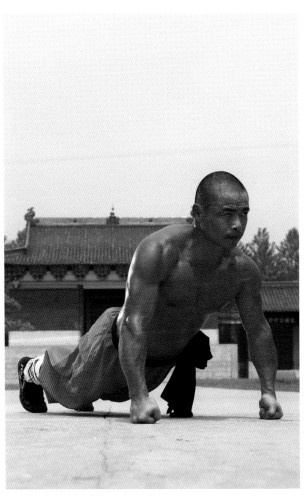

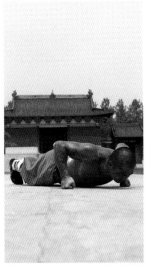

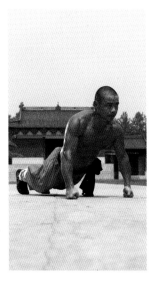

2. Exhale and lower your body down, keeping your back straight, your whole body should be in one long line.

3. Inhale and come up. REPEAT 20 TIMES.

1. Place your hands or your fists onto the floor, the weight of your feet is on your toes. Inhale.

TIE NIU GENDI
METAL COW DIG THE FIELD (QIGONG PRESS UP)

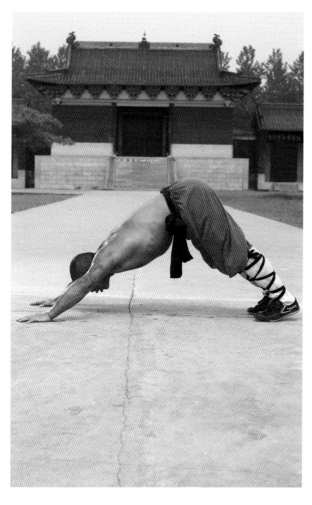

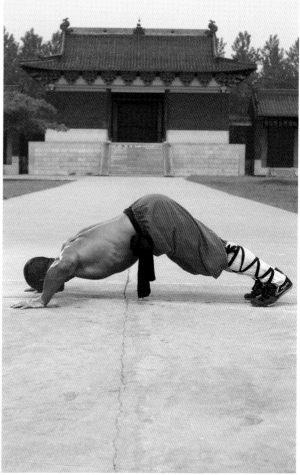

1. Place your hands on the floor and step your feet out behind you. Feel a stretch in your back and your calf muscles. Inhale.

2. Bend your arms and drop your body until it's just off the ground, while slowly moving it forward until it's flat, your body still off the ground.

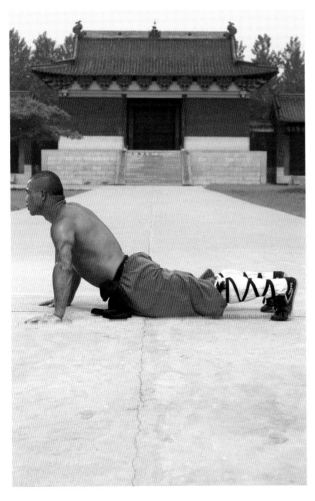 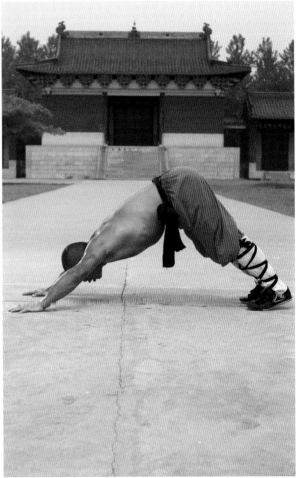

3. Push up from your arms and bring your head back. Exhale.

4. Come back into your first position and REPEAT TEN TIMES.

MA BU SQUAT

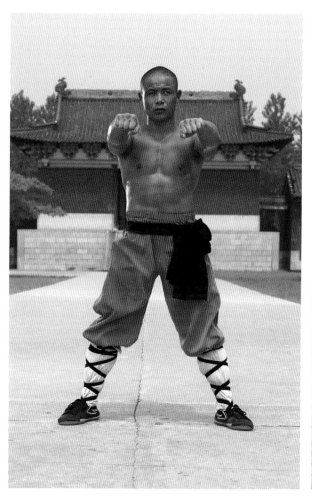 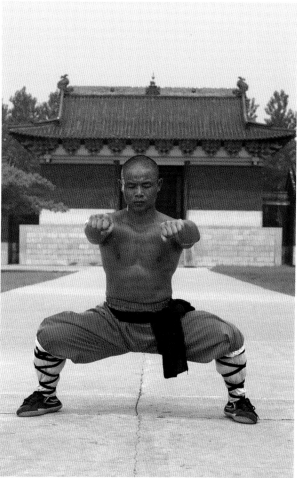

1. Stand with your feet hip width apart, your fists out in front of you. Inhale.

2. Squat into ma bu. Exhale.
REPEAT 20 TIMES.

KNEES UP
RUNNING ON THE SPOT

This simple looking
exercise is surprisingly
challenging. Keep your back
straight. Make sure your
stomach is pulled in.
Run so that your knees
touch your stomach.
REPEAT 100 TIMES.

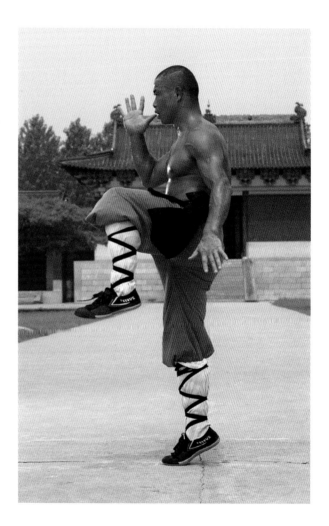

WU LONG PAN DA
BLACK DRAGON HANDS

If you can, start off by practicing close to a wall. This will guide you into how narrow the movement is. It looks like a complicated movement but once you've understood it, it's very easy. Think of it as if you are swimming, you do two strokes of backstroke and two strokes of front stroke. Your whole body moves together to make your body more flexible. This movement relaxes your muscles. The arms don't stop but continue to move so they have momentum until the final movement when you drop into pu bu.

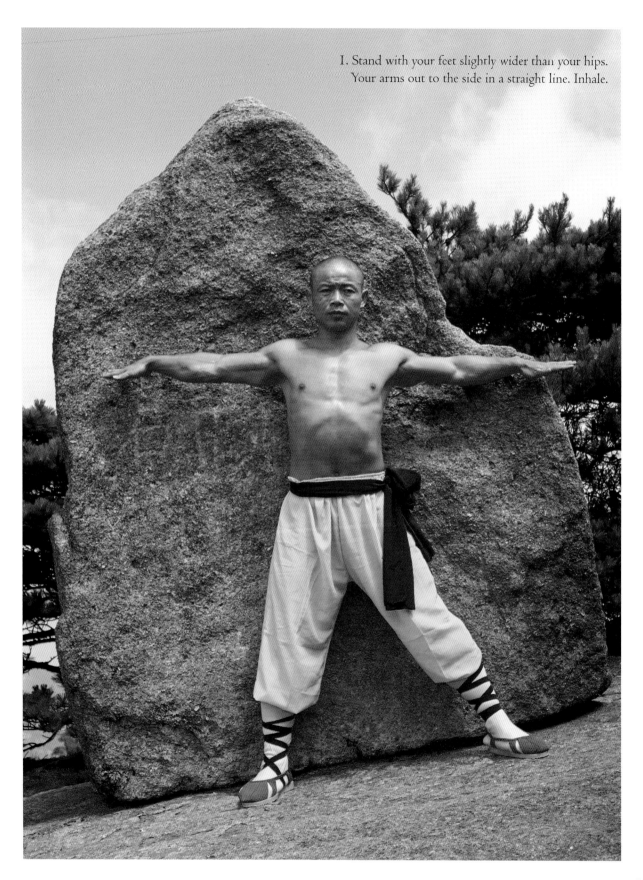

1. Stand with your feet slightly wider than your hips. Your arms out to the side in a straight line. Inhale.

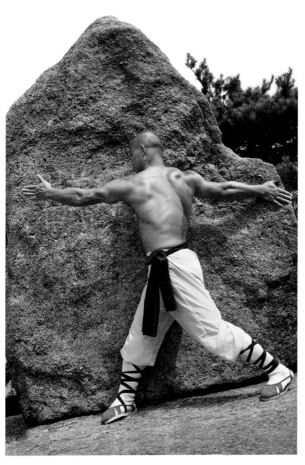 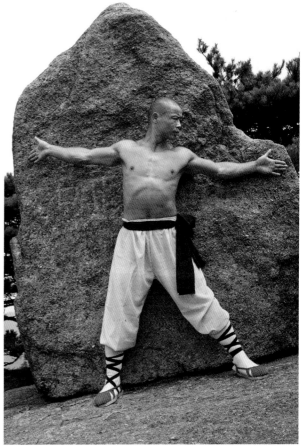

2. Turn your body to the left hand side and move your arms as if you are doing backstroke. The second time you move your arms, come back to the centre.

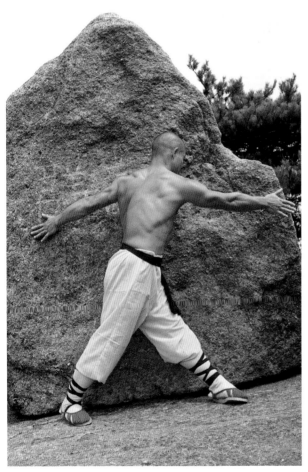

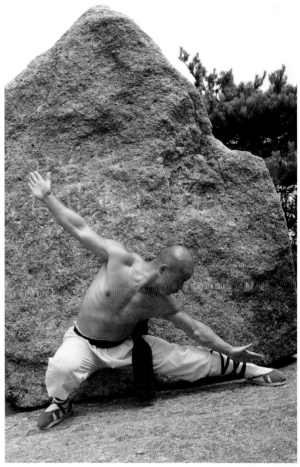

Turn your body to the right hand side and move your arms as if you are doing front crawl, the second time you move your arms go into pu bu. Exhale.
REPEAT ON THE OTHER SIDE. DO 5 ON EACH SIDE.

CHAPTER TWELVE
STRETCHING

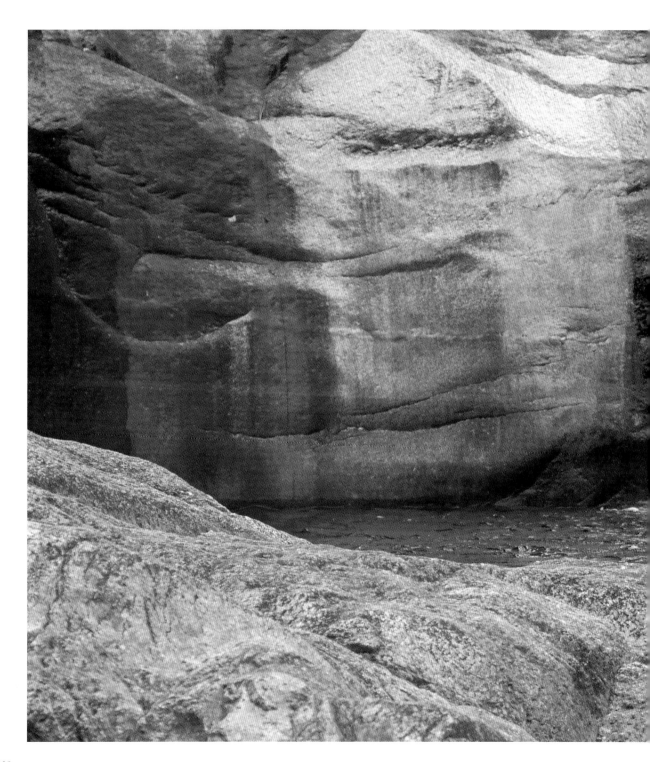

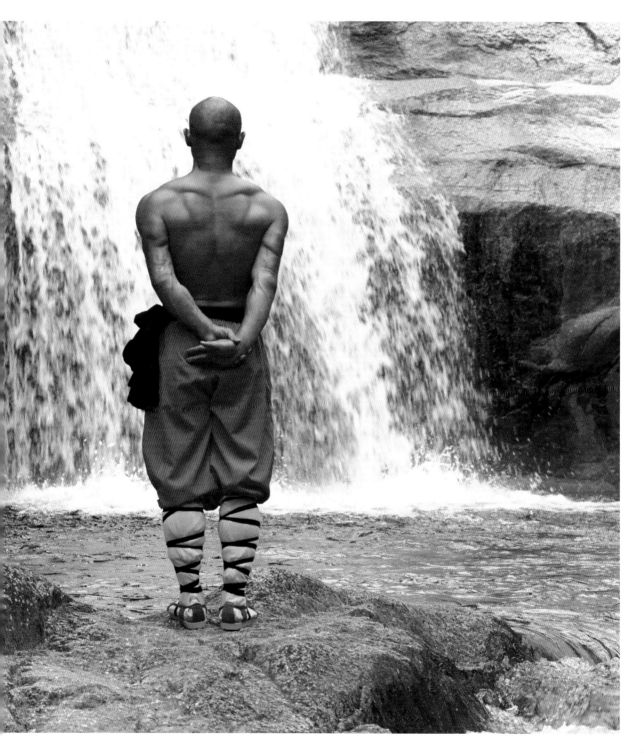

As I mentioned earlier on in the book, if you look at a picture of me stretching please don't feel discouraged. If you are as stiff as a board and your muscles are tight, after you have read the directions let your body move in the direction I am stretching. You will get as much benefit from your stretch as I do from mine and over time you will be surprised how flexible you will become. You don't need to be able to do the splits but you do need to have a certain degree of flexibility to prevent stiffness and to keep the body young. It is good to aim for the splits because it opens the hips and stretches the legs at the same time.

There should be no pain when you stretch but a gentle stretch that deepens as you breathe into it.

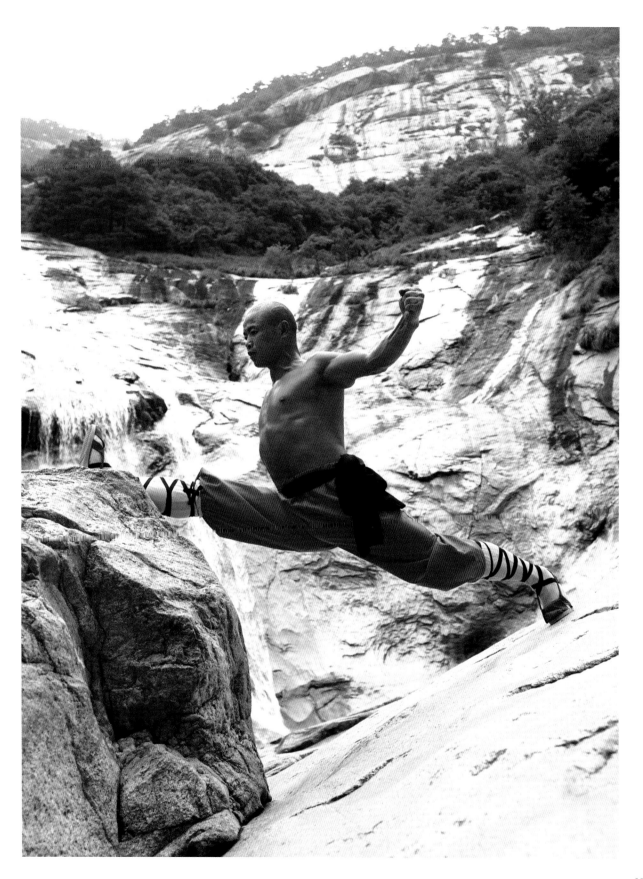

ARM STRETCHES
SHANG LA JIAN
UPPER STRETCH

ZUO LA JIAN
LEFT STRETCH

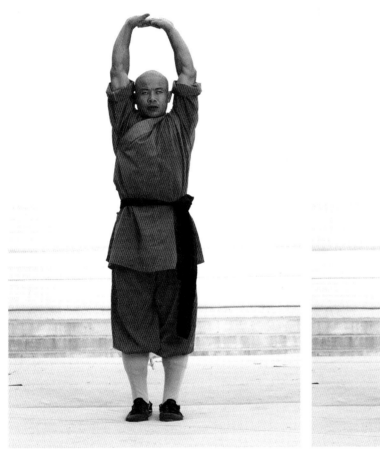 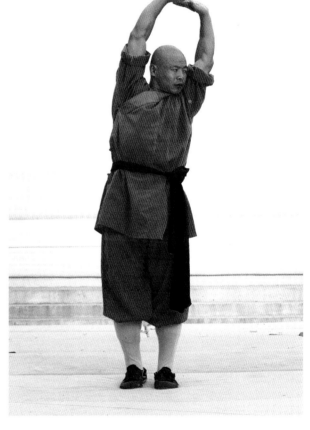

1) Interlace your hands and push your hands up to the sky as hard as you can. Keep your arms straight. Breathe five times.

2) Bend your upper body to your left and stretch your arms as hard as you can. Keep your knees straight. Grab the floor with your feet. Breathe five times.

YOU LA JIAN
RIGHT STRETCH

QIAN LA JIAN
FRONT STRETCH

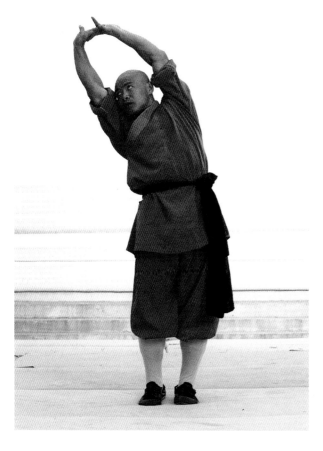

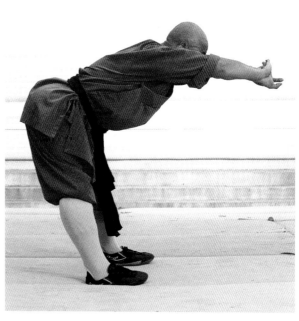

3) Bend your upper body to the right and stretch your arms as hard as you can. Breathe five times.

Use your breath to increase the stretch. Keep your legs straight and your feet rooted to the ground. Your feet need to grab the floor, your back needs to be straight. Focus on your breathing and the direction of your hands. Make a note on the power Move into. . .

4) Open your feet hip width apart, bend at the waist and stretch forward.

Drop your lower back and keep your knees straight. Hands push forward and eyes look forward. Breathe five times.

BAO FO JIAO
HOLD BUDDHA'S FEET

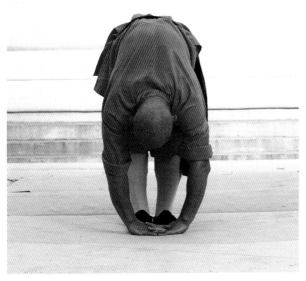

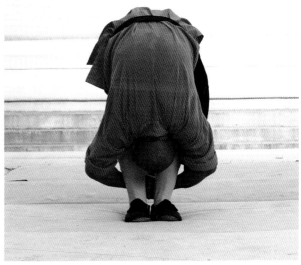

5) Bring your feet together. Drop forward and try to touch the floor with your palms or fingers.
Keep your knees straight. Breathe five times.

6) Place your hands behind your legs and interlace your fingers so your hands are holding your ankles. Place your head on your shin. Breathe five times.
Don't push this stretch and always keep your legs straight. If you can't place your head on the shin don't worry just keep your body dropped and your legs straight and breathe deeply in the stretch. Move into...

LEG STRETCH
ZHENG YA TUI
FRONT LEG STRETCH

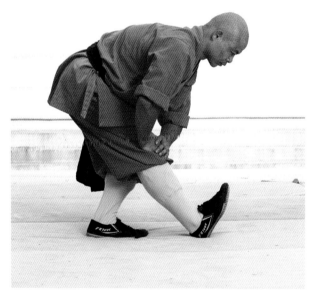
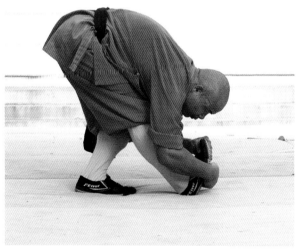

7) Bend your right knee and place your left leg straight out in front of you. Place both hands on your left knee. Lift your left foot onto the edge of the heel. Use your hands to keep your knee straight and stretch your body over your knee. Breathe five times.

8) If you find this easy then clasp your front foot with both hands and try to place your head as far forward as possible. The aim is to touch your feet with your head. Breathe five times.
Don't bend your body but keep it straight.
Change sides and repeat.
Go straight into...

CE YA TUI
SIDE STRETCH

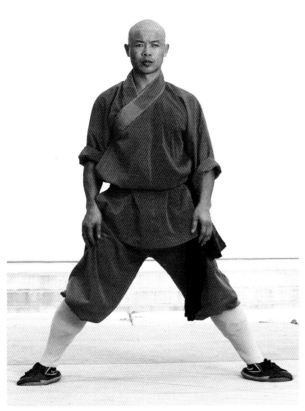
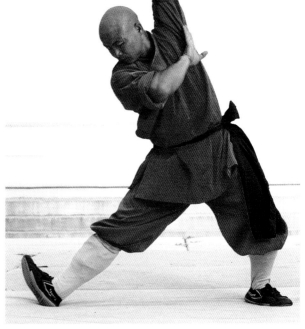

9) Bring your body up and place your legs hip width apart.

10) Raise your left arm over your head and place your right arm across your body. Stretch over to your right, bending your left leg and lifting your right foot so you are balanced on the ball of your foot. Keep your right leg straight and stay in this stretch for five breaths.

11) If you find this stretch easy then lower your body and use both hands to grasp hold of your feet. Hold for five breaths. Eyes look towards the left shoulder. CHANGE SIDES AND REPEAT.

Don't collapse in the lower back but keep your body facing outwards. Feel a stretch through both sides of your body. It's better to stretch high and straight and only progress to movement 11) when you have the flexibility to do so.

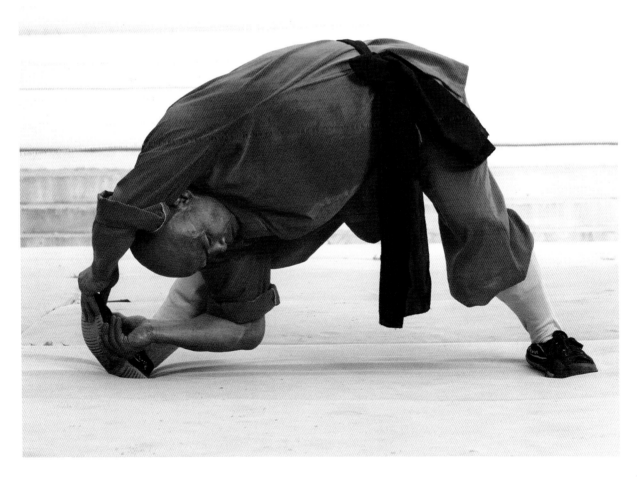

PU BU YA TUI

The next two stretching exercises use two stances from The Five Fundamental Stances, Pu Bu and Gong Bu. Learn the Five Fundamental Stances before doing these two stretches.

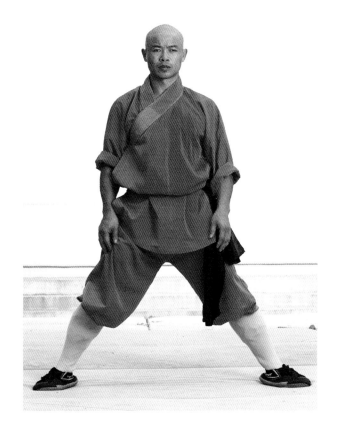

12) Stand straight. Feet hip-width apart.

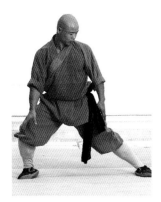

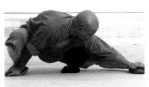

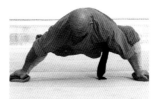

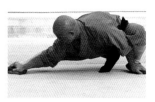

13) Bend your right knee, keeping your left leg straight.

14) Squat down into Pu Bu. Hold your right foot with your right hand and at the same time push out your knee with your elbow so it doesn't collapse inwards. Hold your left foot with your left hand. BREATHE FIVE TIMES.

15) Go into a very low Ma Bu, using both hands to hold both feet.

16) Change to the other side. BREATHE FIVE TIMES.

This exercise opens the hips. Don't worry if you cannot get low at first. The most important thing is to keep your back straight and your hips open, making sure your knees don't collapse inwards. If you can't hold your feet then you can put your hands on your knee.

GONG BU YA TUI

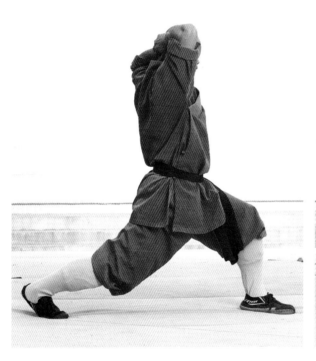 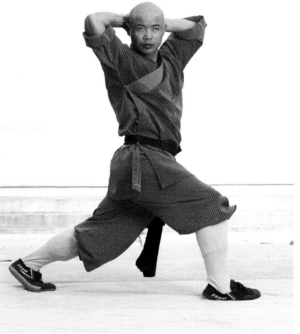

17) Stand up and turn to your left. Go into Gong Bu.

18) Interlace your fingers and place both hands on the back of your neck. Your front foot is flat, push the toes of your back foot and rise up onto the ball of your foot so that you feel a stretch in your calf muscle. Turn your body further to the left to increase the stretch in your leg. HOLD FOR FIVE BREATHS.
Change sides and repeat.
This is a preparation for the splits

SHU CHA
SPLITS

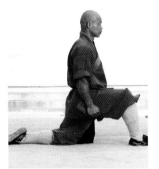

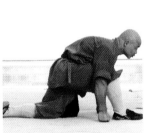

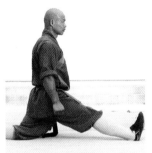

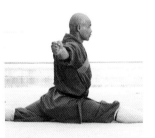

19) From Gong Bu bend your left knee onto the floor. Keep your feet flat.

20) Place your fists on the floor and start to stretch out your back leg.

21) Move your right leg forward by lifting your front foot up. Feel a stretch in your legs. Breathe into the stretch. If you find this easy then…

22) Lift your arms out to the side and move into the splits. BREATHE THREE TIMES AND REPEAT ON THE OTHER SIDE.
Don't push this position. Practise a little every day and you will be surprised how closer you come to the floor.

HEN CHA
FORWARD SPLITS

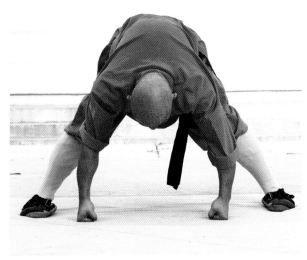

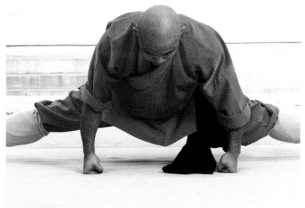

23) Move your body to the centre and touch the floor with your hands.

24) Stretch out your legs and slowly lower them to the floor. BREATHE FIVE TIMES. If you find this easy then…

25) Place your legs flat on the floor. Bring your arms out to the side. Keep your back straight.
BREATHE FIVE TIMES.

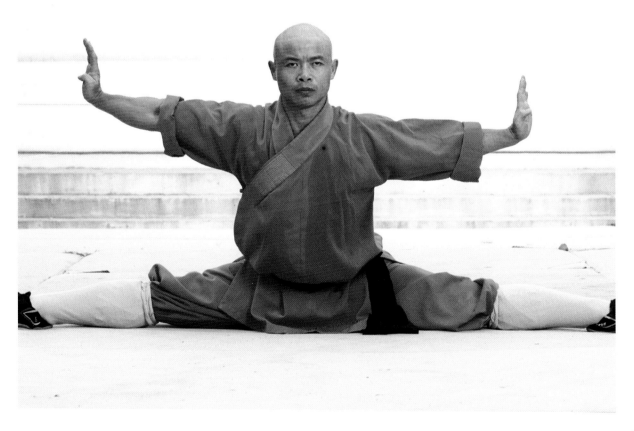

CHAPTER THIRTEEN

FIVE FUNDAMENTAL STANCES

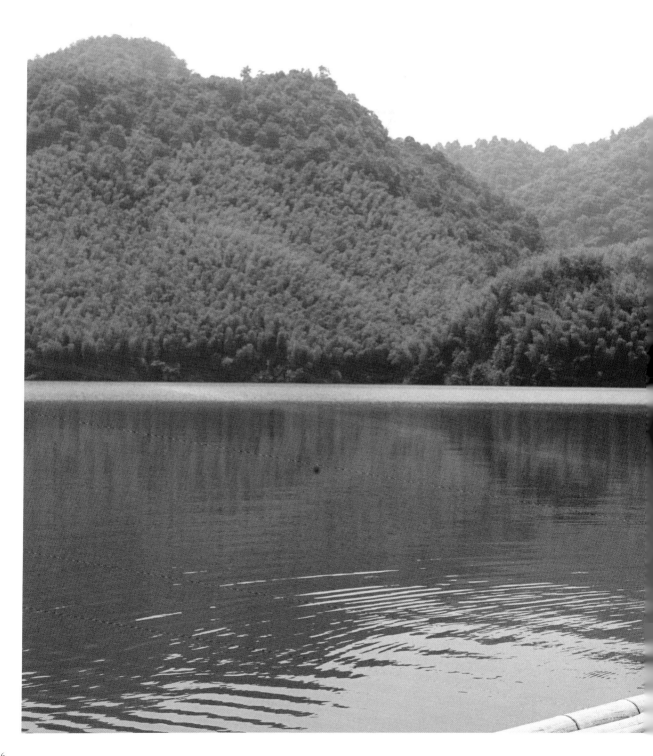

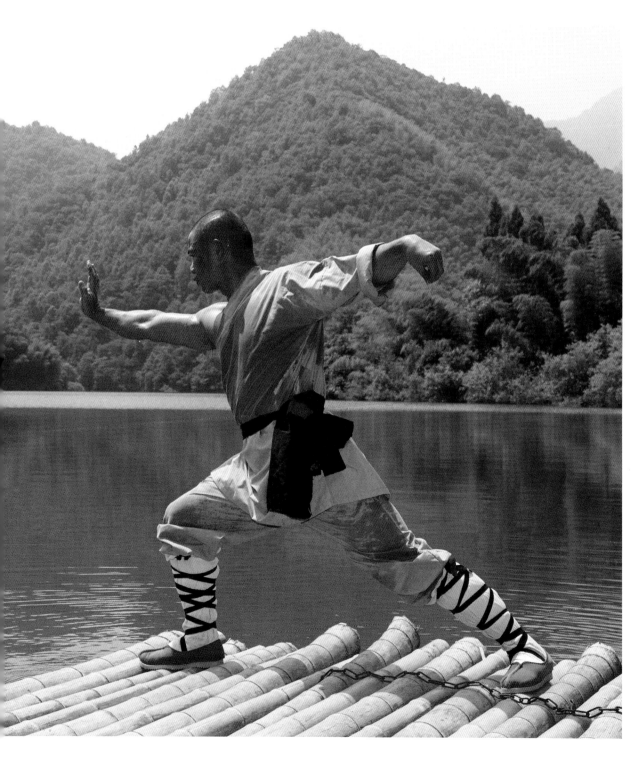

THE FIVE FUNDAMENTAL STANCES:

Are the keys to learning the Shaolin forms
Strengthen your legs
Build your co-ordination and balance

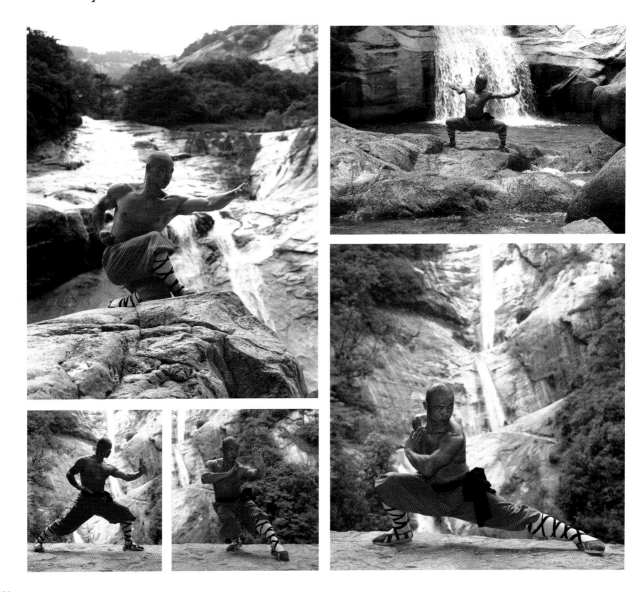

These 5 Stances are the same stances that are in "Instant Health: The Shaolin Qigong Workout For Longevity." All Shaolin forms consist of these five stances, which are then linked together in different combinations. Shaolin Forms are an excellent way to strengthen the legs, and improve balance and coordination. Cyclists and runners strength will improve with the practice of these forms. As martial artists, we hold the forms - this is called static strength. Time yourself and slowly increase the time you hold the stance day by day.

Older people or people with less flexibility should do the stances much higher than me. I do low stances, and all seasoned martial artists should do the same but you will get as much benefit if your stance is high. Listen to your body and work with it.

When you practise the five stances the most important thing is to feel stable in the stances. If you are not stable, this means that when you move on to practice forms your form will not be stable either. When you first begin it is a good idea to check your stance in the mirror. Is your back straight? Is your behind tucked in? Are you grabbing the floor with your feet? Are your eyes focused? Remember - we use every part of our body when we practice Shaolin including our eyes and our mind.

It will take about three months to build the strength of your legs. In some stances, we build up both legs and in other stances we build up one leg or a mixture of the two, with different percentages of weight balanced on different sides. The best way to practise the stances is by staying in each stance for a few minutes and then moving on. Keep the stance as low as you can and, as you get tired, heighten the stance. You can try the opposite way too.

The stances don't just help you to practise your forms, they also build up your will power. If you stay in Ma Bu for two minutes and your legs start to shake, your body wants to stand up and you have to use the power of your mind to push your body to stay a little longer. We call this static stamina because although there is no movement there is effort. When you have finished your stance work, it is a good idea to give your body a shake out or practise some traditional punches and kicks to loosen up any stiffness in the legs. *Make sure the knee - foot alignment is correct. There should be no pain in the knee. If there is then you are doing something incorrectly and need to stop.*

STANDING STRAIGHT

Each of the stances begins with us standing straight, our arms at our side. Our spine should feel long and our chest open with the shoulders relaxed. Our feet are close together with the knees straight but not locked. Allow your hips to roll under a little so the tailbone is slightly tucked in. Check your body for any place of tension and if you find it gently let it go. Your body is now alert, relaxed, focused and ready to go.

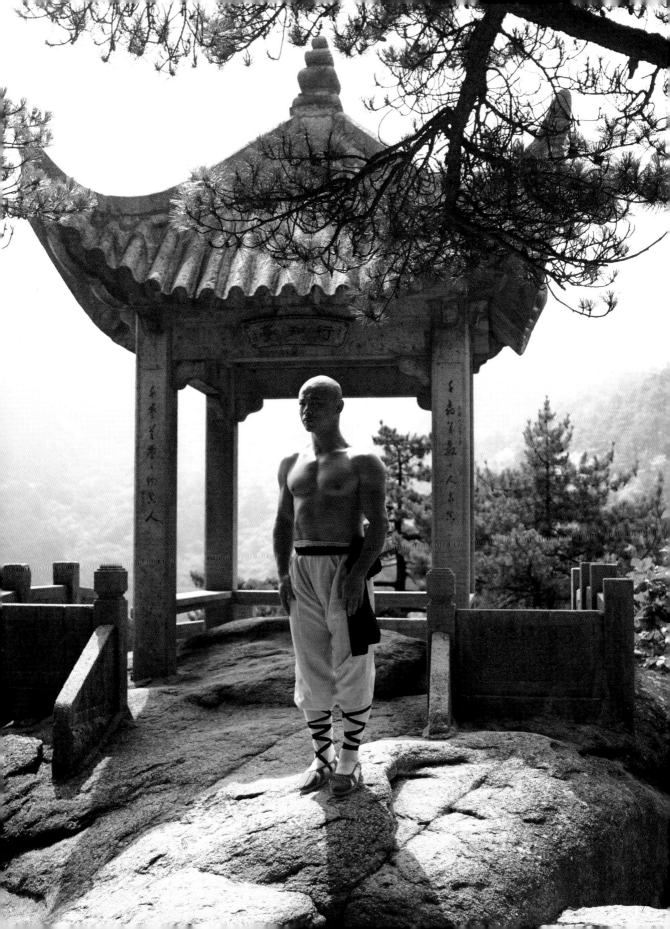

MA BU
HORSE STANCE

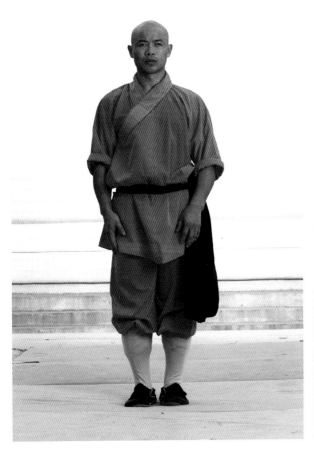

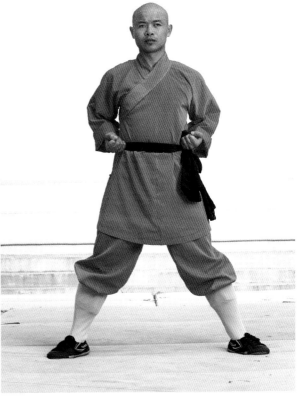

1) Stand straight.

2) Step your left leg out to the side so your feet are wider than the shoulders. At the same time make fists with your hands and draw them into the waist.

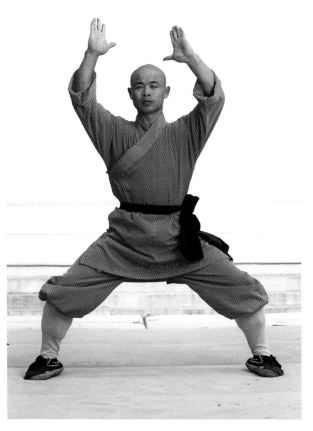
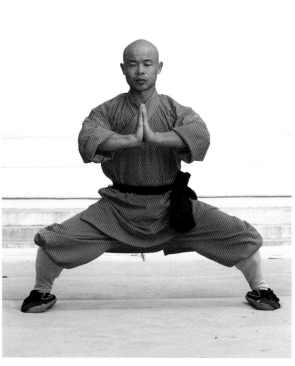

3) 4) Inhale. Lift both hands above your head and bring them down into a prayer position in front of your chest. At the same time squat down into Ma Bu. Exhale.

HOLD FOR 6 BREATHS.

Eyes look forward. Feet grab the floor. Push the knees out a little and don't let them collapse. Tuck your behind in slightly. Elbows go up and wrists go down. Open the chest. Keep the centre of gravity in the middle.

GONG BU

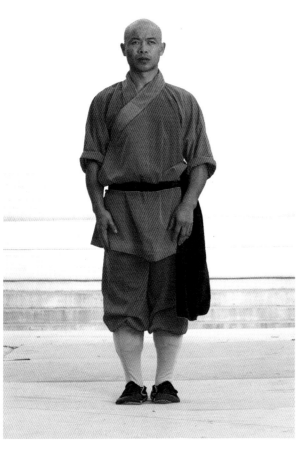

1) Stand straight.

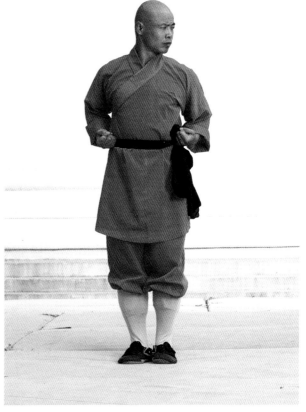

2) Draw your fists to your waist and open your chest. Turn your head to look to the left.

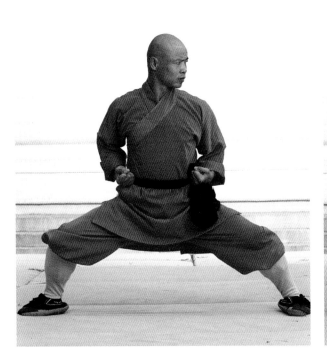 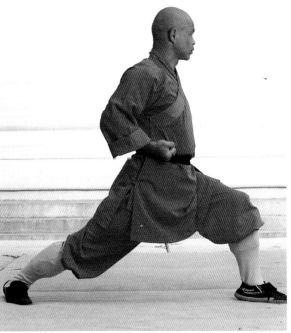

3) Step your left leg out to the side and squat into horse stance.

4) Turn both legs and bend your left leg as much as you can, keeping your right leg straight. Turn your body to face the left.
HOLD FOR 6 BREATHS. REPEAT ON THE OTHER SIDE.

Your right foot should be slightly turned in, it shouldn't be completely straight and needs to be in line with your left foot.

PU BU

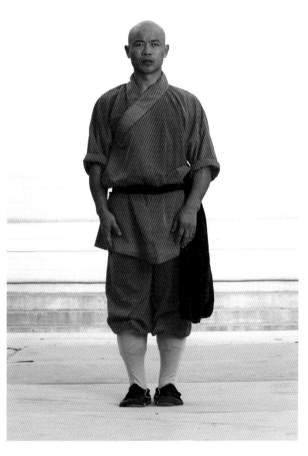

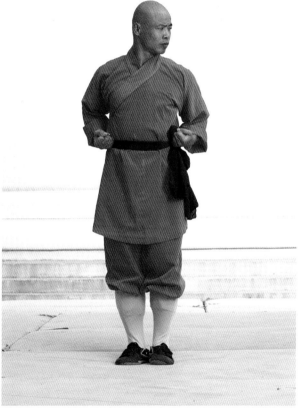

1) Stand straight.

2) Draw your fists to your waist and open your chest. Turn your head to look to the left.

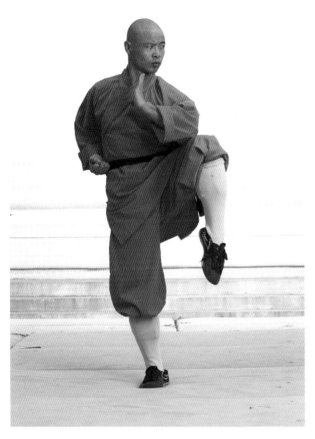

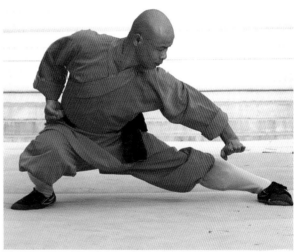

3) Raise your left knee and bring your left hand to your chest.

4) Bend your right knee and squat down until your left leg is straight on the floor. Turn your palm outwards and try to get your palm as close to the left foot as possible.

HOLD FOR 6 BREATHS. REPEAT ON THE OTHER SIDE.

More than 70% of gravity is on your right leg. If you can't place your hand on your foot then place it on your knee or thigh.

XIE BU

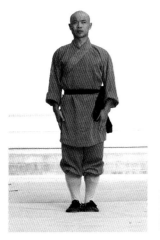 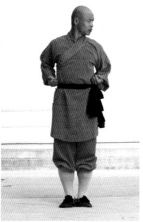 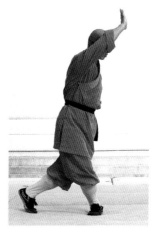 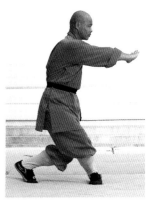

1) Stand straight.

2) Draw your fists to your waist and open your chest. Turn your head to look to the left.

3) Step your left leg behind your right leg. Raise your right hand and bring it across your head as if you are blocking something.

4) 5) Squat down onto your left leg. At the same time your right palm changes into a fist and draws back into your waist.

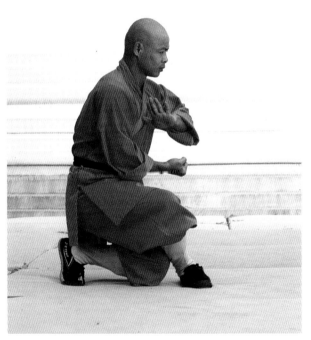 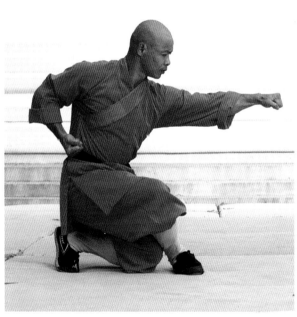

6) Punch out straight with your left hand.
REPS: 3 ON EACH SIDE.

XUE BU

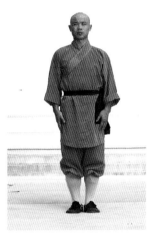 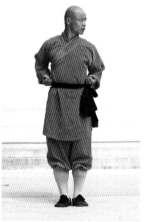 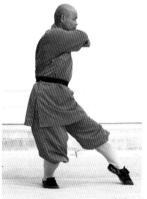 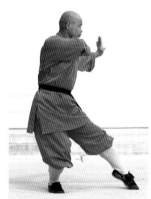

1) Stand straight.

2) Draw your fists to your waist and open your chest. Turn your head to look to the left.

3) 4) Step your left leg out a little to the side. Turn your body and draw half a circle with both hands — your left hand draws a circle in front of your chest, your right hand draws a bigger circle outside your body.

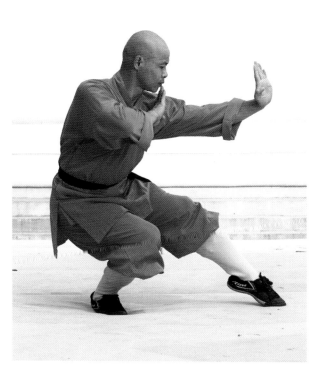

Apart from Ma Bu, repeat the movements on the opposite side. If your left leg is in front it's called "Zhuo Gong Bu". If your right leg is in front it is called, "You Gong Bu". You link these five stances together in Chapter Sixteen.

5) Bend both knees.
HOLD FOR 6 BREATHS. REPEAT ON THE OTHER SIDE.
95% of the weight should be on your back leg. Check by lifting your left leg

CHAPTER FOURTEEN

THE FIVE FUNDAMENTAL KICKS

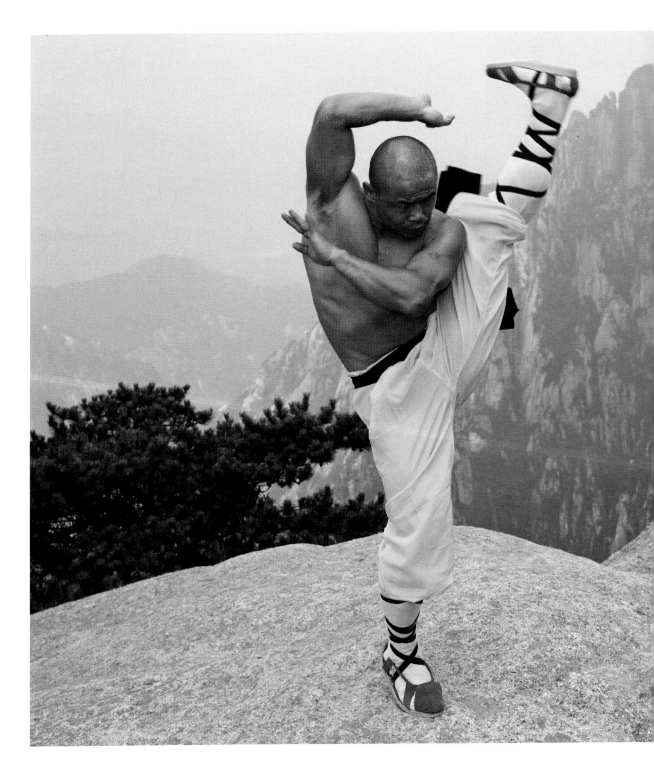

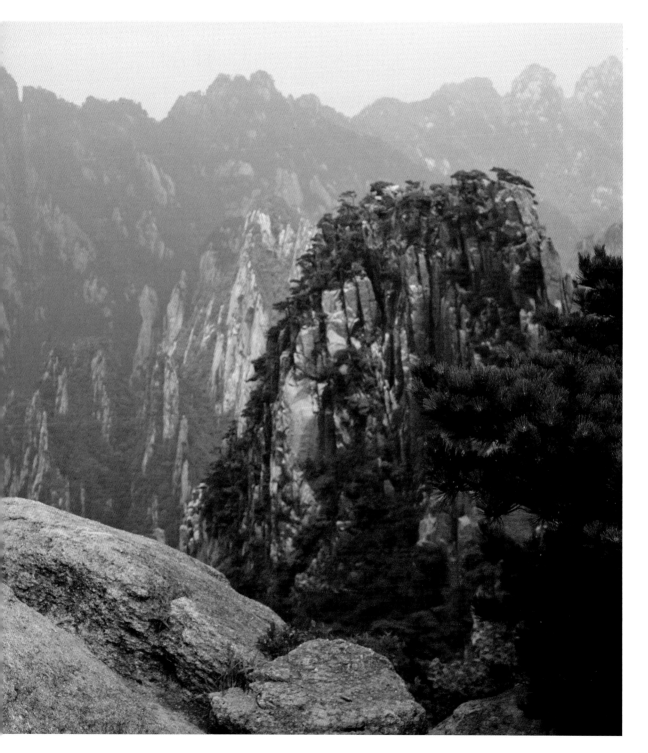

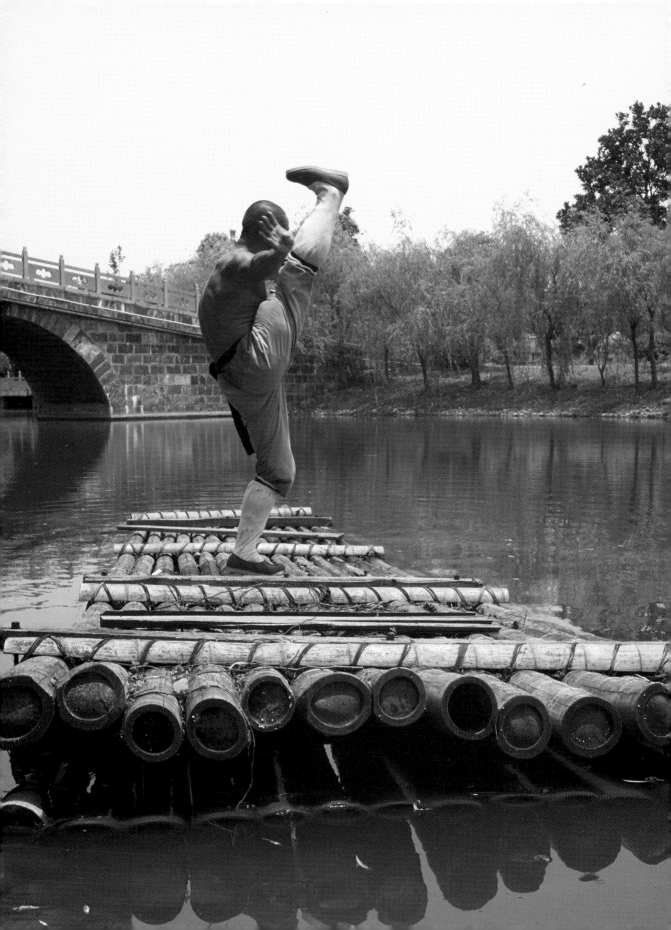

Why are Shaolin Martial Artists so flexible? Because we do dynamic stretching as well as regular stretching.

There is a major difference between the flexibility of a yoga student and the flexibility of a Shaolin student. A Shaolin student has sharpness, power and speed to their flexibility because the purpose of their flexibility is to kick. The Five Fundamental Kicks increase flexibility in the legs and open the hips. I have done these kicks nearly every day of my life since learning them.

Before you do the kicks, you must do the warm up, stamina training and stretching. When you first kick, don't go to the maximum of your flexibility but test your leg, how is your muscle? How are your ligaments? Once you've done a series of kicks in this way, you can then go to the maximum of your flexibility. WARNING: Never do these kicks without warming up first or you will pull a muscle.

It's not important how high you kick but how straight your back and legs are. If you can only kick to your waist, this is much better than kicking a bent leg to your head or bending your back so your kick reaches your head.

BE SURE TO:
1) LOCK BOTH KNEES.
2) DON'T BEND EITHER LEG.
3) KEEP YOUR BODY STRAIGHT.
4) KEEP YOUR ARMS STRAIGHT.
5) REMEMBER TO BREATHE.

ZHENG TI TUI
FRONT KICK

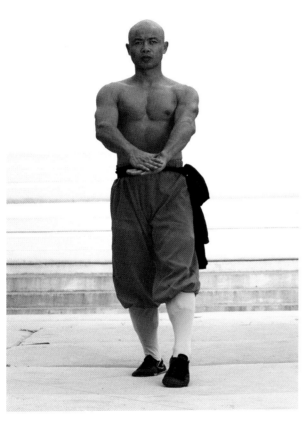 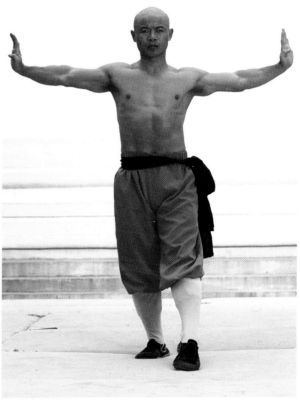

1) Stand with your feet together.

2) Prepare: Slap your right hand on top of your left hand in front of you and at the same time step your left leg forward, using your toes to touch the floor. Then bring your arms out to the side as if you are pushing two walls away from you. Inhale at the same time as your preparation.

3) Keep your arms pushed out to the side and kick your right leg straight out in front of you and towards your head. Exhale on the kick.
REPEAT 10 TIMES THEN CHANGE SIDES AND REPEAT 10 TIMES WITH THE LEFT LEG.

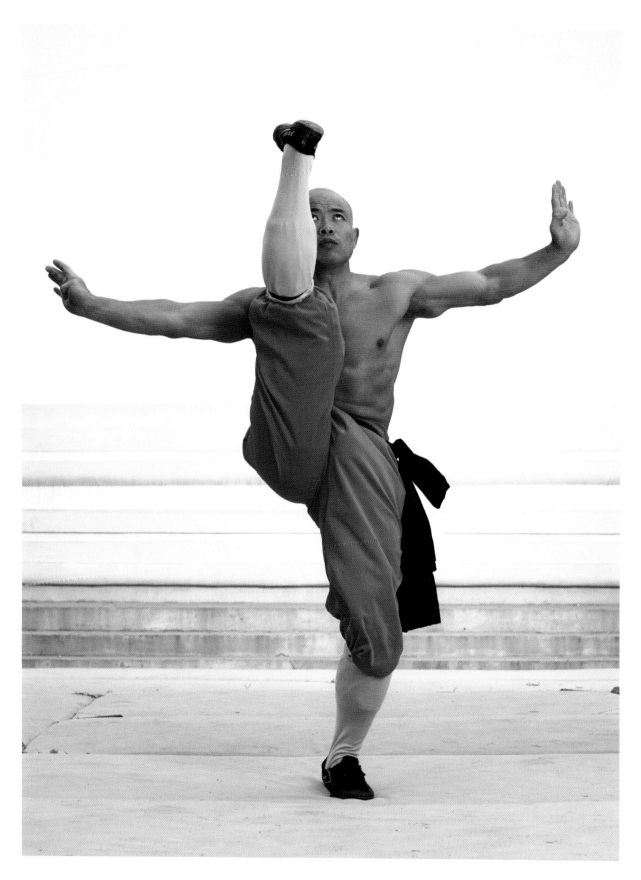

SHI ZI TI TUI
CROSS KICK

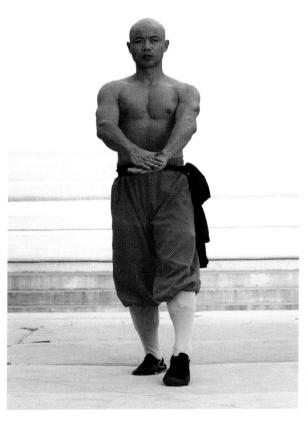
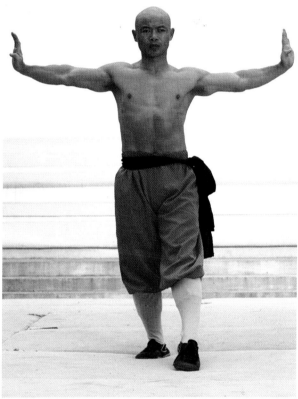

1) Stand with your feet together.

2) Prepare: Slap your right hand on top of your left hand in front of you and at the same time step your left leg forward, using your toes to touch the floor. Then bring your arms out to the side as if you are pushing two walls away from you. Inhale at the same time as your preparation.

3) Kick your right leg across your body as if you want to reach your shoulder. Exhale on the kick.
REPEAT 10 TIMES THEN CHANGE SIDES AND REPEAT 10 TIMES WITH THE LEFT LEG.
(Please note: your supporting leg should be straight. Due to an injury in my leg I can't have a straight leg.)

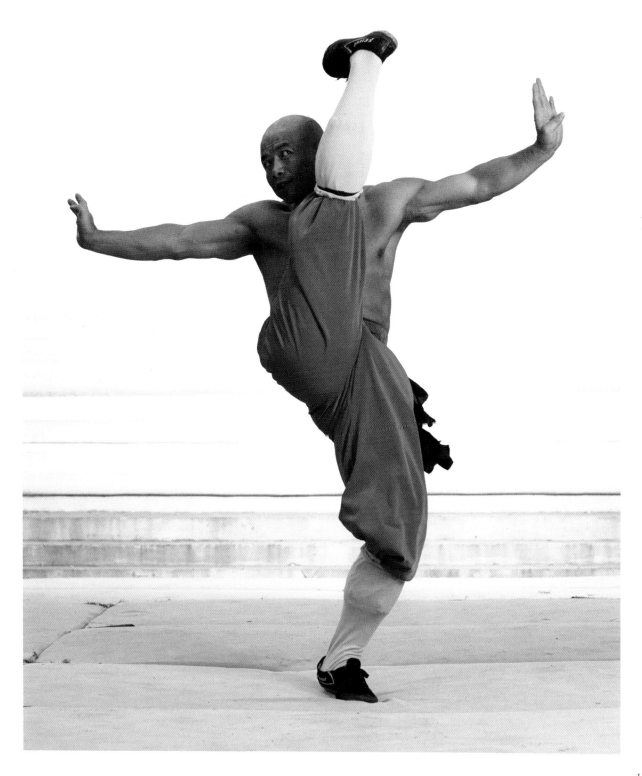

CE TI TUI
SIDE KICK

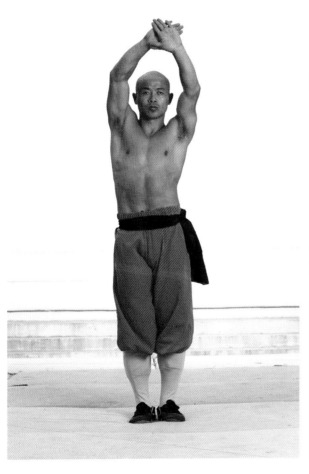 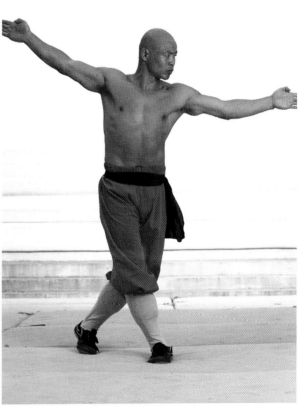

1) Prepare: Turn your head to the left and slap your right hand on top of your left hand in front of you, at the same time step your left leg behind your right leg. Then bring your arms out to the side, your right arm slightly higher than your left arm. Inhale at the same time as your preparation.

2) Kick your left leg out to the side as if you are aiming to kick behind your shoulders. Bring your right arm over your head, and your left arm across your body. Exhale on the kick.

3) REPEAT 10 TIMES THEN CHANGE SIDES AND REPEAT 10 TIMES WITH THE LEFT LEG.

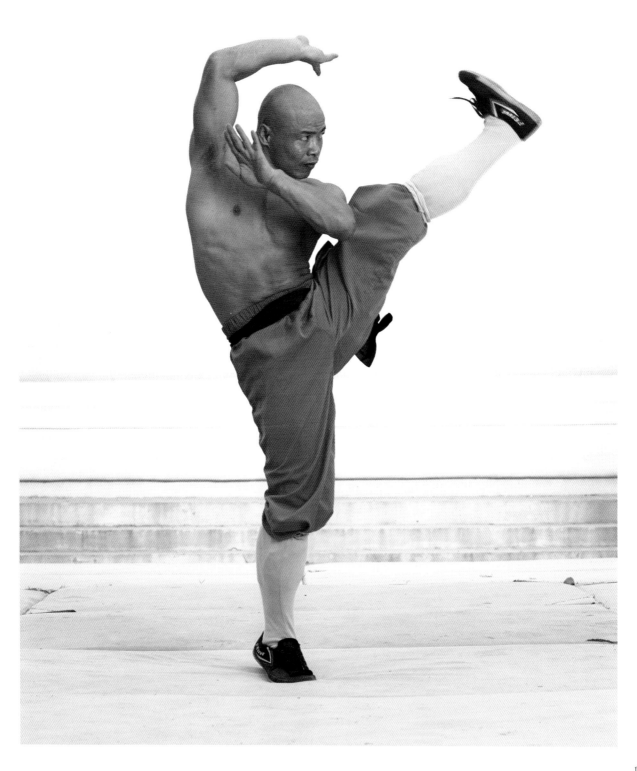

WAI BAI TUI
OUTSIDE KICK

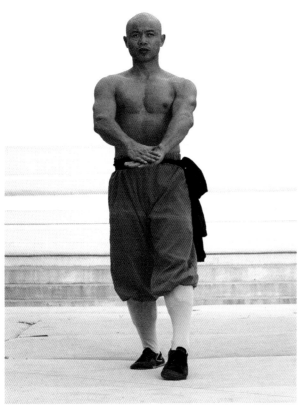 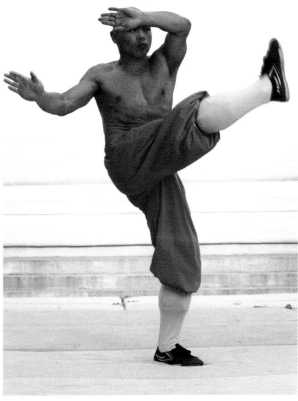

1) Stand with your feet together.

2) Prepare: Prepare: Slap your right hand on top of your left hand in front of you and at the same time step your left leg forward, using your toes to touch the floor. Then bring your arms out to the side as if you are pushing two walls away from you. Inhale at the same time as your preparation.

3) Bring both hands to the right hand side of your body, kick your right leg across your left leg then move your hips so that your leg kicks in a circle, when your leg is at the centre of your body, move your hands in front of you and slap your hands with your feet. Exhale on the kick. Arms go back into the prepare position. *Visualise a half circle, this is the movement of your kick.*
REPEAT 10 TIMES THEN CHANGE SIDES AND REPEAT 10 TIMES WITH THE LEFT LEG.

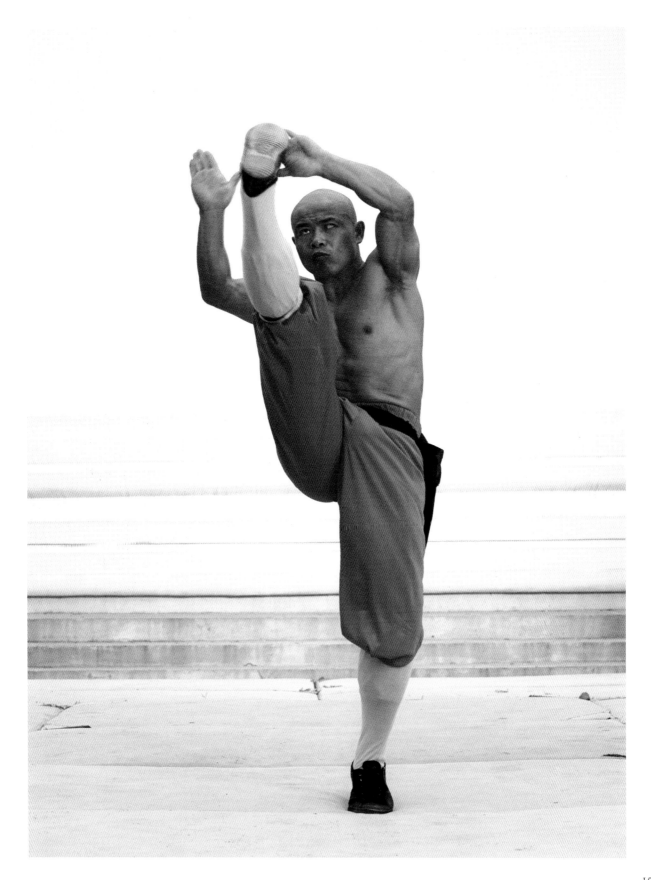

LI HE TUI
INSIDE KICK

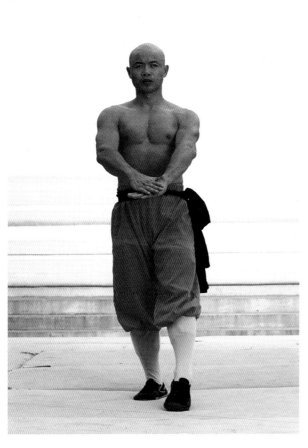 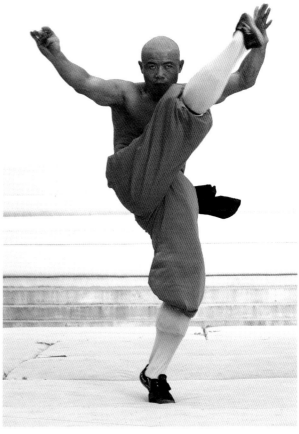

1) Stand with your feet together.

2) Prepare: Slap your right hand on top of your left hand in front of you and at the same time step your left leg forward, using your toes to touch the floor. Then bring your arms out to the side as if you are pushing two walls away from you. Inhale at the same time as your preparation.

3) Kick your right leg out to your right hand side and bring it all the way round in a semi-circle to your left hand side so your foot slaps your left palm. Kick as close to your body as possible. Exhale on the kick. Arms go back into the prepare position.
REPEAT 10 TIMES THEN CHANGE SIDES AND REPEAT 10 TIMES WITH THE LEFT LEG.

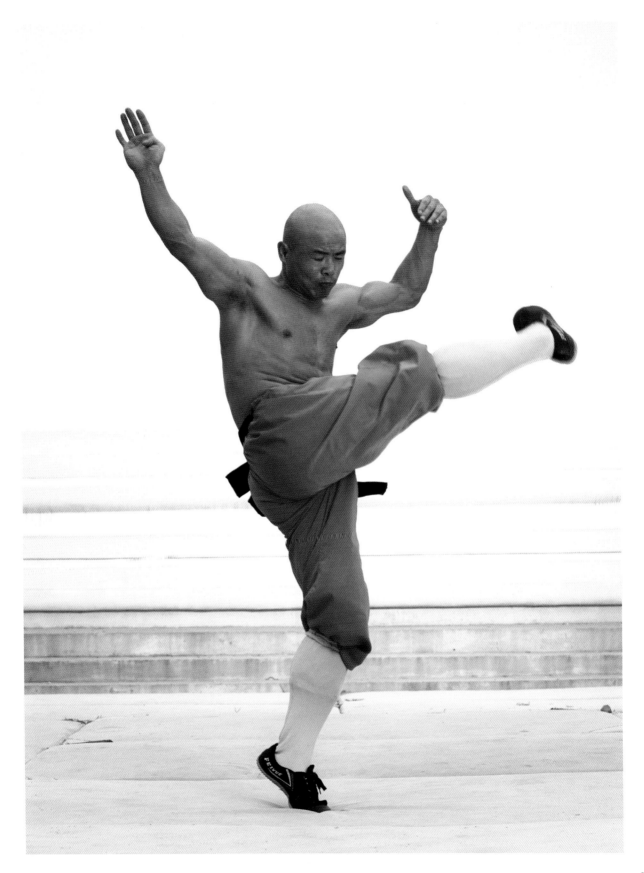

CHAPTER FIFTEEN

SHAOLIN TRADITIONAL PUNCHES

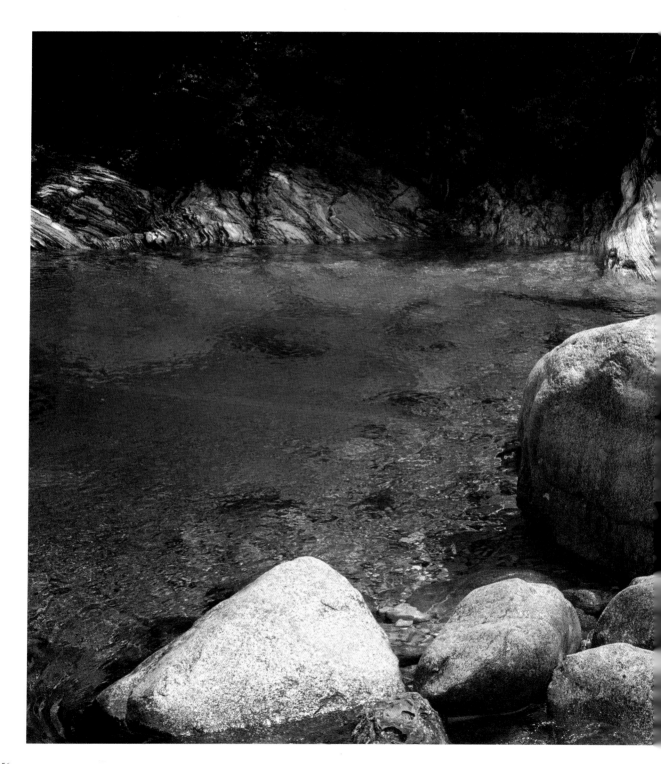

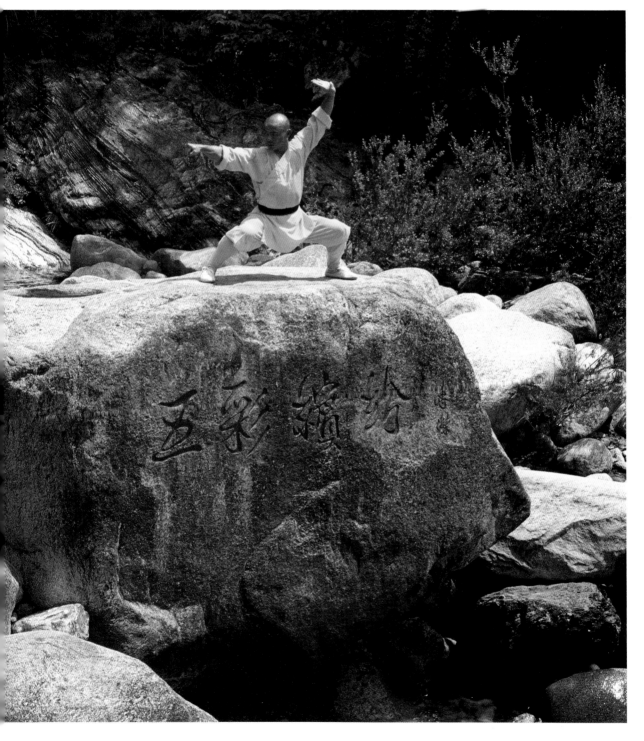

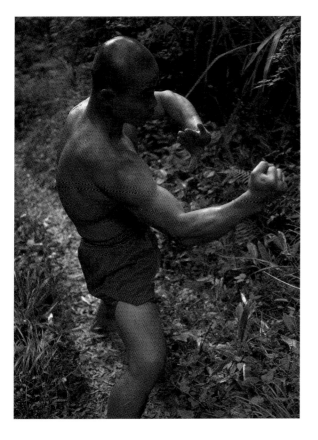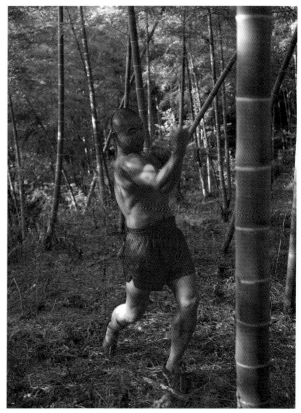

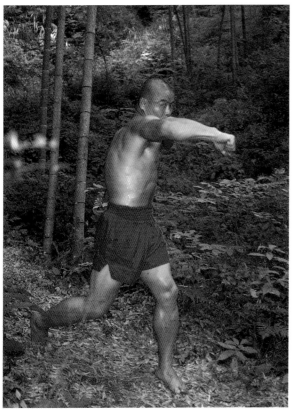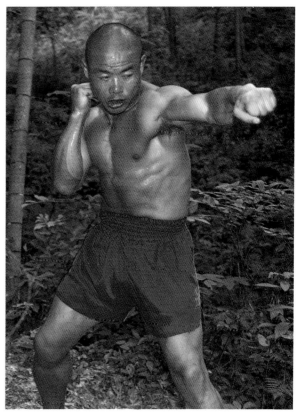

Once you have learned the Five Fundamental Stances you can then move onto the Shaolin Traditional Punches. A great exercise for fighters is to combine these traditional punches with modern punches. The depth of the stance increase leg strength, and the movement makes the hips work so that the whole body moves together. A common pitfall is to use the upper body only to punch, the punch needs to come from the hip.

This is a whole body movement with the body working as one.

Once you have mastered these punches you can then move onto the Shaolin Traditional Forms.

BE SURE TO:
1) USE YOUR WHOLE BODY TO PUNCH NOT JUST YOUR ARMS.
2) MAKE SURE YOUR FEET GRAB THE FLOOR.
3) KEEP YOUR STANCES STABLE, THE LEVEL OF YOUR SHOULDERS SHOULDN'T MOVE WHEN YOU CHANGE STANCE.
4) BREATHE.

MA BU JIE DA

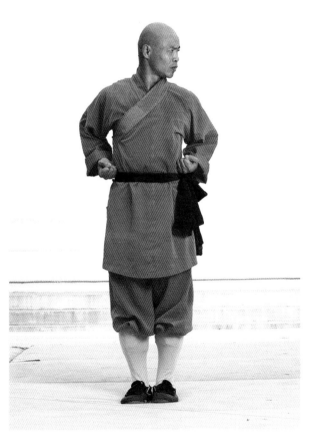

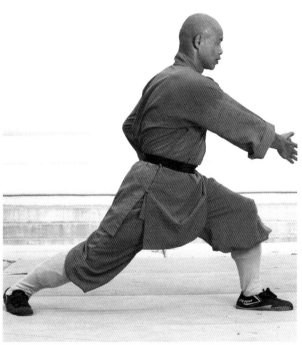

1) Prepare. Stand with both feet together. As you inhale, clench both fists and bring them to your waist while turning your head to the left.

2) Step your left foot out to the side and go into gong bu and bring your right arm over your left leg in a blocking movement.

3) Keep moving your arm until it's over your head and punch your right arm while moving into ma bu, exhale on the punch.
REPEAT 10 TIMES THEN CHANGE SIDES AND REPEAT 10 TIMES ON THE OTHER SIDE.

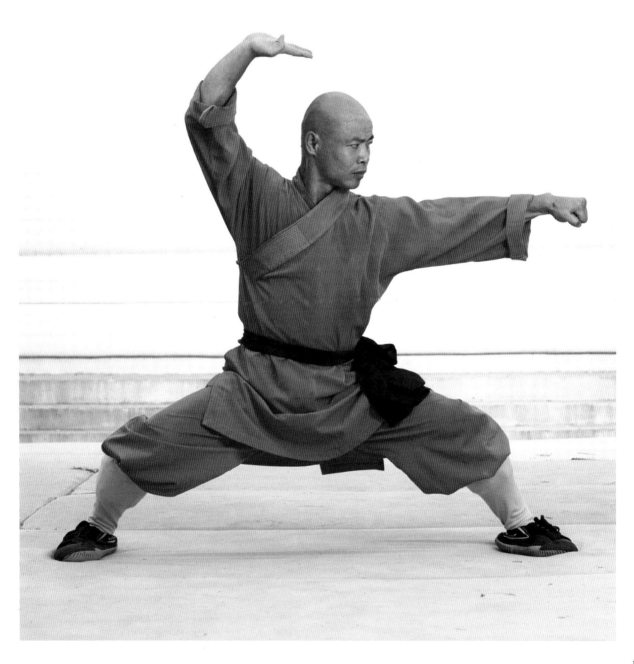

KAI GONG SHI

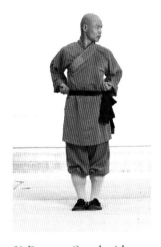 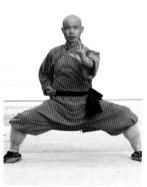 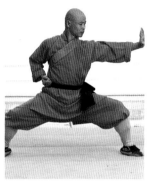 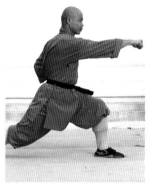

1) Prepare. Stand with both feet together. As you inhale, clench both fists and bring them to your waist while turning your head to the left.

2) Squat down into ma bu and bring your left arm out in front of you, push your palm.

3) Stay in ma bu and move your arm to your left hand side.

4) Move into gong bu and exhale as you punch your right fist and place your left fist on your waist.

5) Move into ma bu as you draw your right arm back as if you are drawing a bow and arrow and punch on the exhale with your left fist.
REPEAT 10 TIMES THEN CHANGE SIDES AND REPEAT 10 TIMES ON THE OTHER SIDE.

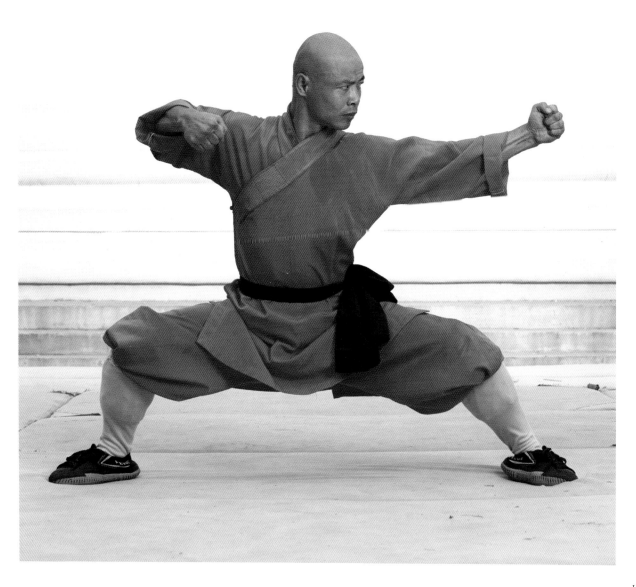

CHAPTER SIXTEEN

SHAOLIN TRADITIONAL FORMS

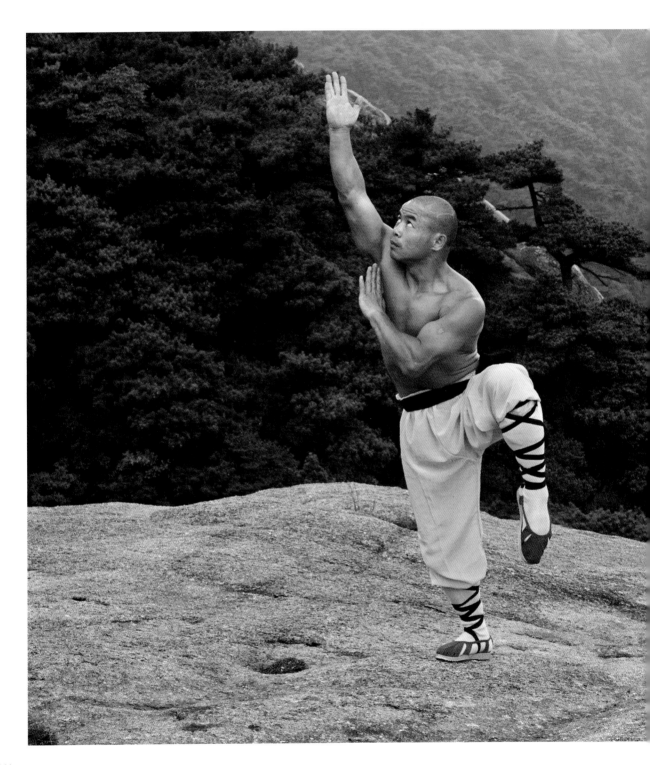

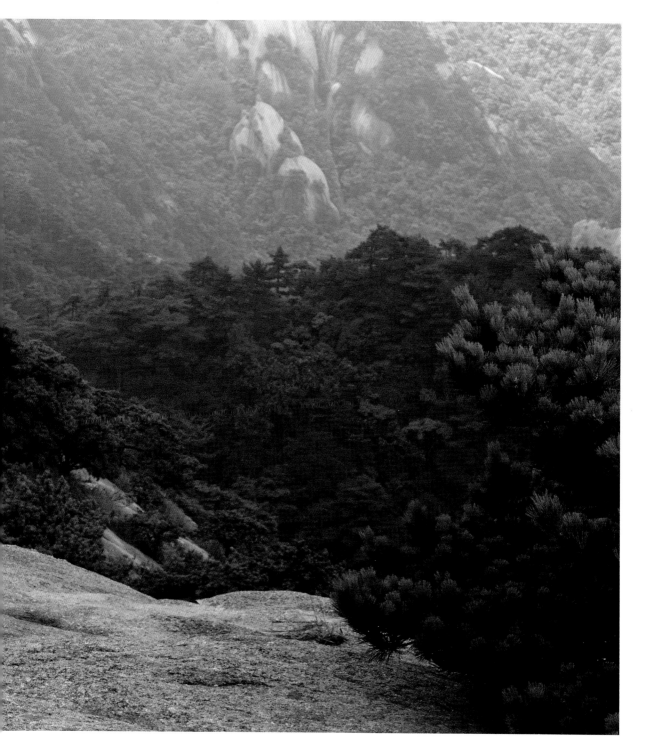

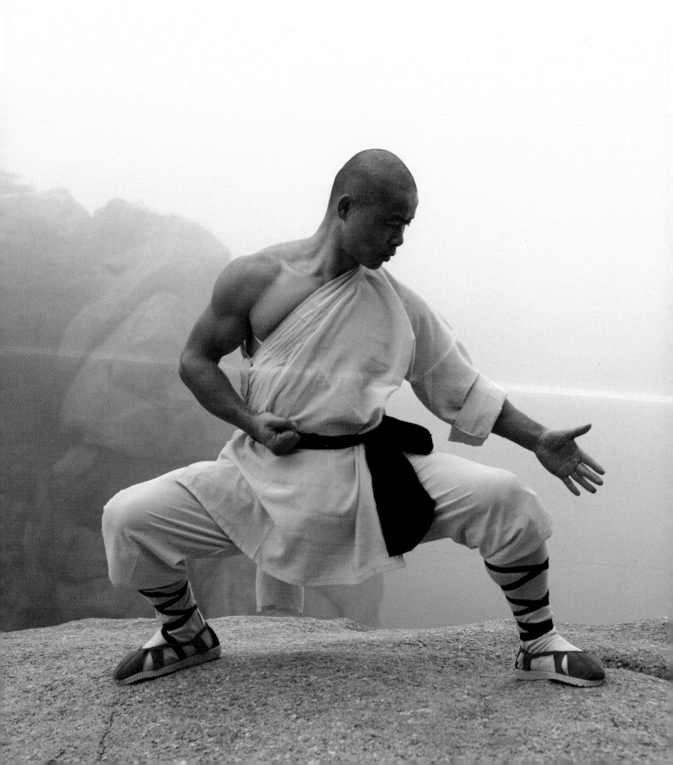

You need to have mastered the Five Fundamental Stances and the Shaolin Traditional Punches before you embark on these forms. You can adjust the stances by making them higher or lower, seasoned martial artists should have low stances. Start off by doing the forms slowly so that your breath and movement are correct.

Your breath and movement should work as one, your breath helps the movement to flow.

Once you've mastered the movements, deepen your stances and quicken the pace of the form.

BE SURE TO:
1) RELAX YOUR BODY
2) KEEP YOUR EYES STRONG.
3) GRAB THE FLOOR WITH YOUR FEET.
4) DO REVERSE BREATHING.

WU BU QUAN
FIVE-STANCE FORM

This form may look easy but it is challenging to move through the stances correctly. If you find it easy, you're doing it incorrectly! This is an excellent form to do as it links the Five Fundamental Stances together like a chain. The first three movement are all done on an exhale and can be practiced separately as a traditional punch combination.

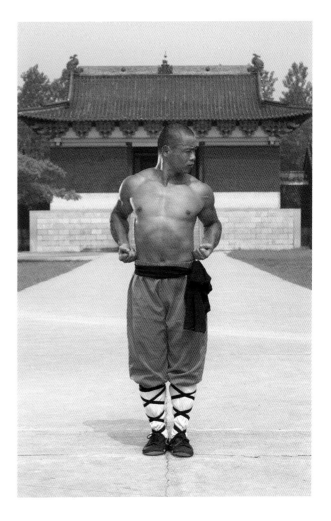

1) Stand with both feet together. As you inhale, clench both fists and bring them to your waist while turning your head to the left.

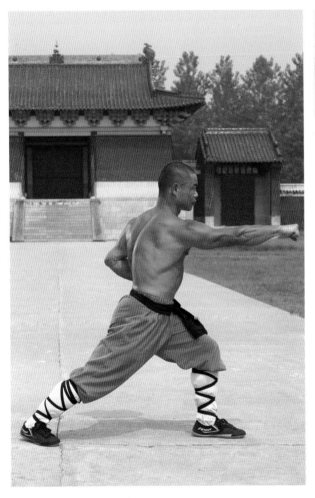 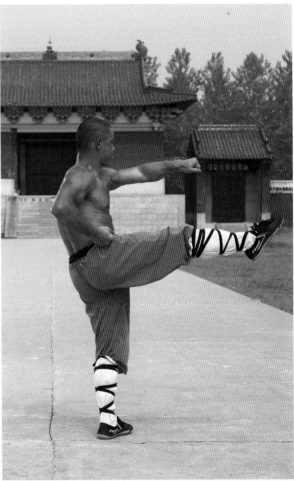

2) Step your left leg out to the side and move into ma bu, your left hands grabs something as if you are grabbing your opponent then you move into gong bu and punch your right fist out in front of you as you exhale.

3) Exhale and bring your right fist to your waist. Exhale and kick your right leg out while punching your left fist straight out in front of you.

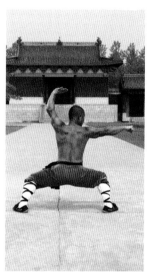 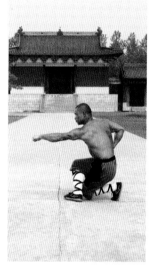 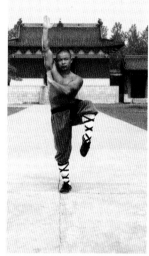 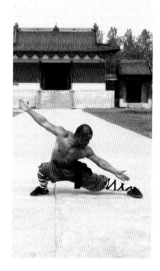

4) Inhale. Drop your right leg onto the ground and go into Ma bu. Exhale, bring your left arm into a block across your face then move it over your head and punch your right fist out to the side.

5) Inhale. Bring your left foot behind your right foot and go into Xie Bu. Exhale, punching your left fist out in front of you, bring your right fist to your waist.

6) Inhale and turn your body to the front, lift your left knee up to your waist, bring your left arm across your body, close to your armpit, and your right arm straight up, both hands are open and not clenched. Your eyes look at your right hand.

7) Exhale as you drop down into pu bu, both arms straight, the right arm higher than the left arm.

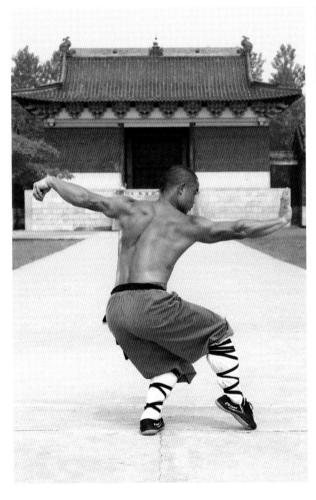 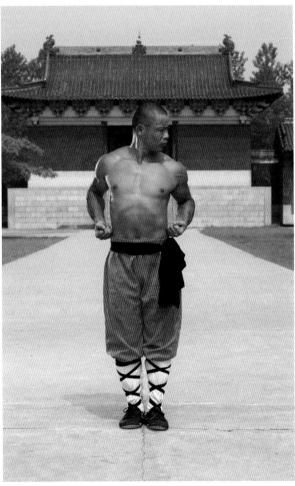

8) Inhale. Stand up and bring your right hand forward, your left hand touches your right palm, at the same time bring your right leg forward. Push your left palm out in front of you and move into xue bu. Your left hand in gao shou (claw). Exhale.

9) Inhale. Turn your body to the front, bring both feet together and both fists to your waist and turn your head to the left.
REPEAT THE WHOLE MOVEMENT ON THE OTHER SIDE.

SI BI QUAN
STAMP BLOCK PUNCH FORM

At the Shaolin Temple this traditional form is taught to top-level disciples because it is so simple. The simplicity makes it harder because you can't hide anything; you need to show the meaning inside the form. It's recommended that you watch Shaolin Workout I where I teach this form.

THIS DECEPTIVELY SIMPLE FORM USES TWO STANCES: MA BU AND GONG BU. IT BUILDS:

STAMINA
COORDINATION
STRENGTHENS THE LEGS
ACTS AS A GATEWAY TO IRON LEG
CENTERS AND GROUNDS THE BODY

In this form you move in four different directions, it is as if you are in a confined room and you are trying to break yourself out of four walls. Imagine a clock on the floor, your feet are at the centre of the clock and you move your feet 9 - 3, 6 - 12, 6 - 3, 12 - 6, 3 - 9 to finish. Each time you are on a line, you do two punches.

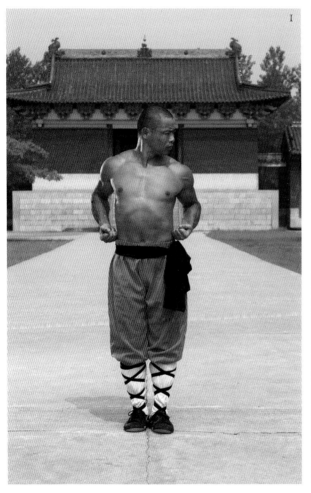
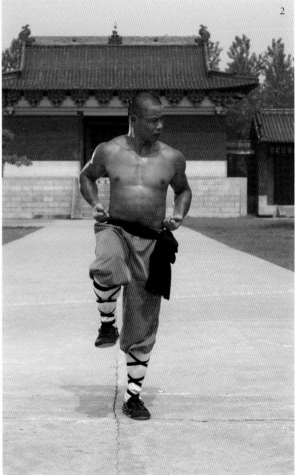

1) Stand with both feet together. As you inhale, clench both fists and bring them to your waist while turning your head to the left.

2) Lift your right leg a little and stamp it onto the ground.

3) Move your left leg to the side and go into ma bu. Chop your left hand across your left knee.

4) At the same time your right hand punches out to the side and you move into gong bu.

7) Bring your right leg back to your left leg.

REPEAT MOVEMENTS 2 - 7 UNTIL YOU ARE BACK WHERE YOU STARTED.

5) Turn your body forward and move into horse stance, bring your right hand over your face and chop it across your right knee.

6) Move into gong bu and punch your left fist.

It takes 10 punches for you to return to your starting position. Once you are back to your starting position:

8) Bring both feet together, bring your arms over your head and inhale.

9) As you bring your arms down exhale.

CHAPTER SEVENTEEN

HOW TO CONTINUE YOUR SHAOLIN WORKOUT

Now that you've mastered the stances, forms, and kicks, you have learned the fundamentals of Shaolin Kung Fu. This is your foundation; it's up to you what you want to make from this foundation. Do you want to continue training in traditional Shaolin? Do you want to move into fighting? Do you want to continue to get stronger and fitter?

If you want to know more about Shaolin, I teach a graded system of Shaolin Qigong and Kung Fu which is available as DVDs and downloads from my website. I also teach a Shaolin Summer Camp in China close to the Shaolin Temple. This is for students who are passionate about martial arts and are happy to train hard. We do three training sessions a day so that the student experiences what it is like to live the life of a Shaolin disciple.

Or you can continue to train at home with the teachings from this book. Now that you know the contents, begin to play with them and vary them, do more kicks on one day, more forms on another day, move from traditional punches to modern punches or traditional kicks to fighting kicks, increase your stamina training by doing more reps. Be creative. The most important thing is to enjoy your training. Training in Shaolin is a positive thing. It sharpens the body and sharpens the mind. Now you are a Shaolin Warrior. Happy training!

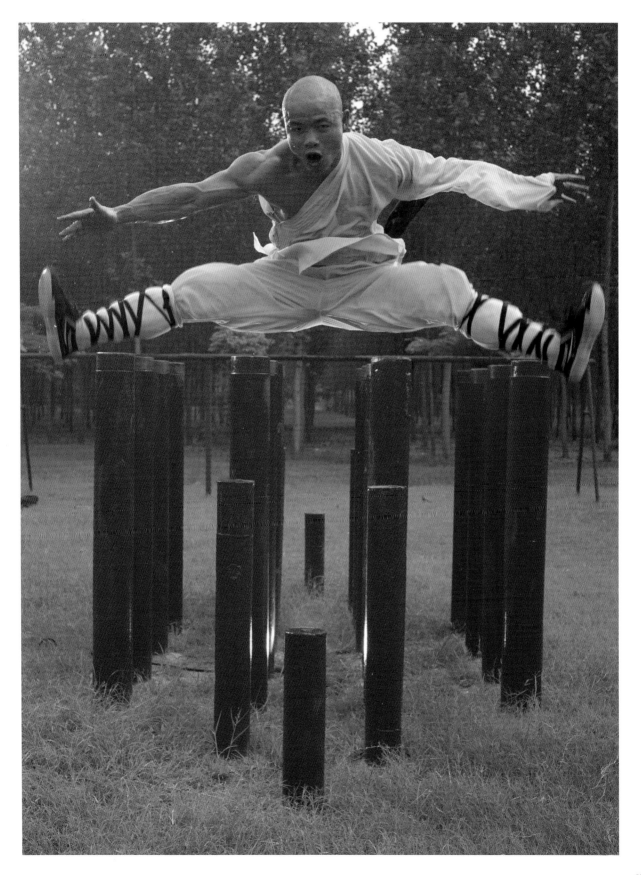

We recommend you purchase

SHAOLIN WARRIOR:
SHAOLIN WORKOUT VOLUME 1

as a compliment to this book. Available from www.shifuyanlei.com

Also in this series

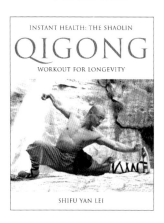

Available as a kindle and on the apple store in the USA and UK

Available from www.shifuyanlei.com and all good book stores.

SHIFU YAN LEI'S
SHAOLIN WARRIOR TRAINING GROUP

This is a Facebook group for people who train with my books, DVDs, and downloads.

WWW.SHIFUYANLEI.COM

Here you can access lots of free content and videos on Shifu Yan Lei's blog page, Twitter, and YouTube.
You can also download or buy Shifu's Shaolin Warrior series, which offer a graded path to Shaolin.
The bamboo and metal brush is available for Qigong massage.